What physicians are saying about **YOUR MIND AND BREAST DISEASES:**

"An illuminating book that must be read by every woman in America and her physician." JOSEPH BO-HORQUEZ, M.D., Director, Division of Radiation Oncology, S.U.N.Y. Downstate Medical Center, Brooklyn, N.Y.

"I have found this book an excellent presentation of the breast cancer problem written from the point of view of a woman who had lesser surgery. Her insights into medical practice are startling and revealing. Doctors should read the book to help them understand the feelings and motivations of their patients." BERNARD GARDNER, M.D., Director of Surgical Oncology, S.U.N.Y Downstate Medical Center, Brooklyn, N.Y.

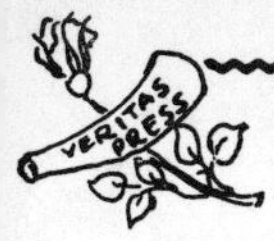
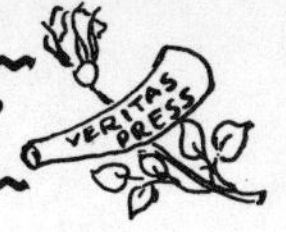

Your Mind and Breast Diseases

(A psychologist-breast cancer patient who did not have a mastectomy describes her experiences and discusses the relationships between the mind and breast diseases)

by

Sarah Splaver, Ph.D.

VERITAS PRESS • New York, N.Y. 10467 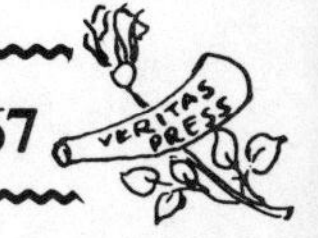

Published by VERITAS PRESS,
3310 Rochambeau Ave.,
New York, N.Y. 10467

Library of Congress Catalog Card No. 78-62152
ISBN 0-932208-00-2

this book is dedicated

to

my breast specialist

without whom this book could not have been written

— another physician the likes of him it's impossible to find —

CONTENTS

No coward soul is mine,
No trembler in the world's storm-troubled sphere:
I see Heaven's glories shine,
And faith shines equal, arming me from fear.

Emily Bronte.

FOREWORD

With insight, sensitivity and dramatic force, Sarah Splaver uncovers myths about breast cancer, exposes some cruel medical practices and reveals some humane and effective ones, and inspires us to struggle against cancer in general and breast cancer in particular. She demolishes the myths and helps the reader to face a malignancy with courage and the will to live. And she does this with wit, humor and the force of facts.

Dr. Splaver's is the voice of a champion for *human* rights in the treatment of women with breast cancer.

If you want to empathize with a woman who has breast cancer, if you want to experience vicariously the vicissitudes of the words, "It's malignant," and you want this reported by an experienced counselor and author who has both personal and researched knowledge about it, read Sarah Splaver's YOUR MIND AND BREAST DISEASES. When a woman has a malignancy in her breast, Dr. Splaver points out with the clear voice of reason, FACT not FEAR must prevail to enable the woman to make the wisest choice, and she alone, the author says, armed with those facts and the will to live, should make that choice.

This book has the power of a documented exposé in the tradition of Lincoln Steffens and the spirit of life and determination in the tradition of Helen Keller. Dr. Splaver is the David come to battle with the Goliath of breast cancer, and once again David is victorious.

Milton Schwebel, Ph.D.
Professor, Graduate School of
Applied and Professional Psychology,
Rutgers University

Part One

The Major Myths Must Be Demolished

THE MAJOR MYTHS MUST BE DEMOLISHED

Your mind and your breasts are interrelated and interconnected. Your mind reacts when something acts on your breasts. Similarly, your breasts may react when something acts on your mind. If you are stricken with a breast disease, you must make your mind work to your advantage.

You can — and must — imbue your mind with a positive attitude and positive outlook and with a determination to fight back. Your mind will then help you not just to live, but to live effectively.

I heard the words, "it's malignant," in the summer of '75. When you hear these words, they shake you up a bit — generally more than "a bit" — and you may wonder how much longer you will be alive. But, you must call upon your mind to help you. You must call forth all of your psychological resources, all of your emotional strengths, and fight back. If you do, you will increase the chances of your living out your normal life span.

On July 14, 1975, I had a tylectomy (popularly called a "lumpectomy") performed on me, in which a small malignant tumor was removed from my left breast. In Part III of this book, I describe some of the weird, funny (strange as it may seem) and not-so-funny personal experiences I have had from that time forward.

After my tylectomy, I embarked upon intensive and extensive investigations into the world of breast cancer. Among my many unanticipated findings are the several myths surrounding the subject of breast cancer. These myths have been repeated so many, many times that they are all too often accepted as fact, although they are fiction.

There are five basic major myths and they all must be exposed and demolished. All women — and men too — are vulnerable to breast cancer. Your life and your breasts may hinge on the exposure and demolition of these myths.

The five major myths are the following:

Myth #1: Breast cancer is a death sentence.
FACT: NO, IT IS NOT! Breast cancer is curable, if it is detected early.

Myth #2: The rich and the famous get the best surgical treatment.
FACT: NO, THEY DO NOT! More often than not, they get the worst. They are more apt to be subjected to more major, more excessive and more unnecessary surgery than the rest of us.

Myth #3: If you object to having a mastectomy, you are neurotic.
FACT: NO, YOU ARE NOT! The woman who has no objection to having a mastectomy is neurotic. The woman who objects has inner emotional strength and self-esteem as a woman and is *not* neurotic.

Myth #4:   The woman who has radical surgery demonstrates courage in doing so.
FACT: NO, SHE DOES NOT! It is fear, not courage, that causes her to
           have radical surgery.

Myth #5:   Every breast malignancy requires radical surgery.
FACT: NO, IT DOES NOT! Every breast malignancy does not require radical
           surgery. With early detection, where the tumor is small and conditions
           are conducive, lesser surgery and/or radiation therapy may be suf-
           ficient and the breast cancer patient's life can be saved and her
           breast(s) may be spared.

When the medical profession does not know the cause of or the best mode
of treatment for a specific illness — as in the case of breast cancer — myths
arise. Breast cancer is a very mystifying illness. When an illness mystifies, the
myths multiply and can do much mischief.

Now, let us examine individually the five major myths surrounding breast
cancer.

Myth #1:   Breast cancer is a death sentence.
FACT: NO, IT IS NOT! Breast cancer is curable, if it is detected early.

Breast cancer is *not* a death sentence. Life is a "death sentence," since
we all ultimately die. Breast cancer and skin cancer are the most curable cancers
and are not and should not be considered "death sentences."

The leading cause of death in the United States is heart disease. More than
750,000 people died of heart disease in this country in 1977. Less than half
that number, approximately 350,000 people, died of cancer in 1977; this number
includes all of the many different types of cancers. Yet, heart disease is
rarely, if ever, referred to as a "death sentence."

Since so many women who had mastectomies have told me that they consider
breast cancer a "death sentence," let us examine *death*.

What is death? Think about this question. Don't come up with a simplistic
answer. Don't say, "It's the end." It may very well be "the beginning"
rather than "the end." It may be the start of a new type of life.

Henry Wadsworth Longfellow put it beautifully when he said:
    "There is no death!
    What seems so is transition;
    This life of mortal breath
    Is but a suburb of the life elysian,
    Whose portal we call death."

Death is a reality of life which we all must face. I faced death at a very
young age. I am the youngest of a family of seven children. When I was a
little girl, the oldest of the children in my family, my older sister, slipped while
crossing the street. The truck driver did not see her. And, thus was terminated
the life of a beautiful, creative, artistic young woman in her early twenties.

Death, to me, meant not just seeing everyone I loved crying hysterically,
but, perhaps even more important, it meant never again being able to have the
company of and being able to look up to my oldest sibling, whom I loved for

the span of years between myself as the youngest and my sister as the oldest made me look upon her as almost a second mother.

For a child, death is a frightening phenomenon. I did not use the words "death" or "died" until I reached college, until I had achieved a certain degree of maturity. Before that, I said someone had "passed away." I could not accept that dreadful, dastardly devil "death" that had brought such tragedy to my parents and other members of my family and had taken my sister from me. At college, I studied philosophy, physiology and psychology — an excellent combination — and became more understanding of my orthodox Jewish parents' views of an afterlife and the Biblical dictum, "Thy will be done." And, death no longer frightened me.

Today, I believe not only in an afterlife, but also in reincarnation. Death does not frighten me at all. For that reason, life is very precious to me. I have found that those who are afraid of death are not truly alive, for their fear of death prevents them from truly living. They are not only afraid of death, they are also afraid of life. I live each day to the fullest. I am neither afraid of life nor of death.

What about you? Does the word "death" frighten you? Why? You are not a child. You are — at least chronologically — an adult. Who told you that breast cancer is a "death sentence"? Why?

I have found that those who succumb to the myth that "breast cancer is a death sentence" are women who have never truly lived, who are afraid of life. I hope you are truly alive, for if you are, you will not be afraid of death. The more afraid you are of death, the more apt you are to become a victim of radical surgery, of excessive surgery.

If you are not afraid of death, you will not succumb to this myth. If you do not succumb to this myth, you will be less apt to become a victim of radical surgery, of excessive surgery.

So many women often say, "How should I kill time today?"

Have you ever said that? If you have, then what you really said is, "How should I be dead for part of today?"

Time is life. If you "kill time," you are dead during that portion of time — that portion of life — that you have "killed."

Living is not just breathing in and out, working at home or elsewhere, and performing certain basic bodily functions. That is *existing,* not *living.* Living is assuming commitments. It is accepting the challenges of life — and life has many challenges. It is facing up to life — and not running away from it. It is aiding those less fortunate than ourselves. It is taking reasonable risks for the benefit of others and ourselves.

Is there something that needs to be done — perhaps to help someone in need — do you do it? If you don't, you aren't really and truly alive. Do you have commitments? Do you accept challenges? Do you take risks? Do you participate in aiding the ailing, the aged, the needy? If you don't, you are quite dead.

Start living — start doing — start helping others. Start accepting challenges; start taking reasonable risks; start participating. Then, you will be alive — and, then, you will not be afraid of death — and you will not succumb to this myth.

Some mastectomees (women who had the surgical procedure known as "mastectomy" call themselves "mastectomees") have told me they believe they are "terminal cases." I have asked them if their physicians had told them this. Invariably, they said, "No," but that they personally "feel like a terminal case."

Actually, we are all "terminal cases" from the moment we are born, for someday our lives on this earth will "terminate." The mastectomees who view themselves as "terminal cases" are in the throes of a state of depression and should get professional help.

I implore all surgeons: when you believe a mastectomy is necessary, do not just surgically "prep", but also psychologically "prep" the patient for this mastectomy. The patient should also be psychologically "prep"ed before she is permitted to leave the hospital. Supportive psychological counseling should be made available to the patient for as long thereafter as necessary.

The mastectomy is a traumatizing, devastating surgical procedure and professional psychological counseling can be very effective in tempering the trauma, easing the emotional devastation, and aiding the patient to adjust to her altered physical state.

We all have much more psychological strength than we bring forth and utilize. To cope with and conquer breast cancer, we must call upon and use these inner psychological resources. Depression prevents a person from doing this. I, therefore, urge all breast cancer patients — those who had mastectomies and those who did not — who view breast cancer as a "death sentence" to get professional help immediately.

We all surely know cases where physicians said patients would die that day or in a day or two and the patients are alive and well five and ten and twenty and even more years later — and the physicians may be gone. Recently, I spoke with a man who is well and active; eighteen years ago, I stood at his hospital bedside and heard a team of six doctors declare that he would die that night! I have been told that several members of that "team" are long gone.

Breast cancer is a strange and mysterious illness. The human body is a wonderful mechanism. When the mind helps it, the body joins the mind in fighting to conquer breast cancer. Several physicians have told me of patients of theirs who had biopsies of their breast tumors a number of years ago. These biopsies indicated that their tumors are malignant. These women refused to permit mastectomies to be performed on them — nor would they permit any surgery at all — and, strange as it may seem, these women are well and living normal, active lives — with their malignancies within them! This is known as *symbiosis*.

Symbiosis is a state in which two diverse types of living matter exist together in harmony. Thus, the cancerous tumors of these women and their normal, noncancerous tissues and organs are living in a symbiotic state. Some may wonder why this happens in some women and not in others. Where it does happen, the mind and the body working together have succeeded in conquering the onslaught of the cancerous body cells. Personally, I would not want a cancerous tumor to remain within me; I would want it to be removed via lesser surgery (lumpectomy).

No, breast cancer is not a death sentence. Breast cancer is curable. Many books have been written on the subject of breast cancer. I have read most (perhaps all) of those written within the past decade and there is only one that I can recommend highly. This is the excellent book entitled, EARLY DETECTION: BREAST CANCER IS CURABLE, written by the world renowned breast specialist, Philip Strax, M.D. Note that Dr. Strax included the phrase, BREAST CANCER IS CURABLE, as part of his book's title.

They MYTH is: Breast cancer is a death sentence.
The FACT is: Breast cancer is not a death sentence. Breast cancer is curable, if it is detected early.

Myth #2:   The rich and the famous get the best surgical treatment.
FACT: NO, THEY DO NOT! More often than not, they get the worst.
          They are more apt to be subjected to more major, more excessive,
          and more unnecessary surgery than the rest of us.

It is a myth, strange as it may seem at first glance, that the rich and the famous receive the best surgical treatment. Among the many things I found, in all the research and investigating I have been doing since I was stricken with breast cancer in July 1975, is that the brainwashing of the public by the traditionalist surgeons with the myth that every breast malignancy requires radical surgery is so pervasive that even the rich, the famous, the celebrities, the persons in the highest levels of government, and even some women who are highly educated (but highly ignorant about their own bodies) have succumbed to this brainwashing. As a consequence, the rich and the famous are more often subjected to major, excessive and unnecessary surgery than are other people.

Some years back when I started counseling, I counseled the children of very wealthy parents. It was then that I first learned, much to my surprise, of how gullible are the wealthy when it comes to matters of health care. They, all too often, believe that the more you pay the better is the medical and surgical care you receive. The more the physician or surgeon charges them the better, they think, he (or she) is, whereas the amount the physician or surgeon charges has little or nothing to do with his (or her) knowledgeability or competence.

The rich tend to believe that with money they can buy the best of everything. This is definitely not so in the realm of surgery.

We have fee-for-service surgery. The more they cut, the more the surgeons get paid — and the rich and the famous have the money to pay for "more." Surgeons may charge whatever they wish, based essentially on the size of the patient's purse and the amount of surgery performed. The rich and the famous have more money than the rest of us and, therefore, they are more apt to be subjected to MORE MAJOR, MORE EXCESSIVE, AND MORE UNNECESSARY SURGERY than the rest of us.

Simply because someone is rich and famous does not make that person knowledgeable about breast cancer. Sad to say, I have found among this class of people so very many who are so very ignorant about their own bodies.

In the case of breast cancer, the rich and the famous generally have radical surgery performed on them, even if lesser surgery or non-surgical treatment would have been just as effective or perhaps even more effective. Rare indeed is the rich and/or famous woman who has had a simple mastectomy, wedge resection, tylectomy, or only radiation therapy, despite the fact that her malignancy may have called for nothing more than any one of these modes of treatment.

The rich and famous mastectomees may smile for the camera, but you do not see them when they sit depressed and shed copious tears in the privacy of their own homes. The public does not see and is rarely aware of the bitterness these rich and famous mastectomees harbor toward the middle-class breast cancer patients who may have had lesser surgery and/or radiation therapy rather than the radical surgery which they had.

A NOTE OF WARNING: I would like to offer these words of warning to all the rich and famous, as well as the middle-class, readers of this book. If you read in the papers or magazines of breast surgeons who performed radical surgery on the breasts of rich and famous women, you would do well to stay away from these surgeons. In the main, these surgeons have gotten into the bad habit of doing excessive and, at times even, unnecessary surgery.

A NOTE OF ADVICE: The rich and famous should fight to abolish fee-for-service surgery and to establish one fee for all types of breast surgery. If there were one fee for breast surgery, whether that surgery be lesser surgery or radical surgery, the rich and famous would have as good a chance of having lesser surgery as any other woman.

The MYTH is: The rich and the famous get the best surgical treatment.
The FACT is: More often than not, they get the worst. They are more apt to be subjected to more major, more excessive, and more unnecessary surgery than the rest of us.

Myth #3:   If you object to having a mastectomy, you are neurotic.
FACT: NO, YOU ARE NOT! The woman who has no objection to having a mastectomy is neurotic. The woman who objects has inner emotional strength and self-esteem as a woman and is *not* neurotic.

The woman who objects to having her breast(s) amputated is *not* neurotic. She is well adjusted and has wholesome feelings of self-worth as a woman.

Let me concisely explain what we mean by the terms "neurosis," "neurotic," "psychosis," and "psychotic."

A neurosis is a behavior disorder that results from the inability of a person to cope adequately with her (or his) emotional problems. The neurotic is in a constant state of stress. A psychosis is a state of being mentally ill. The psychotic has lost touch with reality. The neurotic finds it difficult to cope with reality; the psychotic has fled from reality.

To add a little touch of humor here, let me tell you a tale that is popular among mental health professionals when they are asked to differentiate between neurotics and psychotics. They say: neurotics build castles in the air, psychotics move in, and psychiatrists and psychologists collect the rent.

The person who is neurotic does not have the ability to adjust to stressful situations. She (or he) is forever plagued by feelings of emotional fatigue, fear and inferiority. The neurotic is generally in a state of anxiety. Anxiety is chronic, intense worry.

The woman who permits a mastectomy to be performed on her is in a neurotic state. She is intensely worried and the anxiety continues to build. She is frightened and the fear keeps mounting. She has become depressed and full of feelings of inferiority. Her feelings of inferiority have reduced her feelings of self-worth and self-esteem as a woman, feelings the seeds of which were probably within her prior to her being stricken with breast cancer.

The woman who objects to having radical surgery and says, "No," to the surgeon who advocates radical surgery for every woman with a breast malignancy is well adjusted — *not neurotic* — and capable of coping with stressful situations. She has strong feelings of self-worth and self-esteem as a woman. She has respect for her breasts, her body, her life, and because she has respect for life and a desire to live, she will ask questions and not permit anyone to frighten her into radical surgery.

Some mastectomees have told me that they were told in advance by their surgeons that they needed a radical mastectomy. Some told their surgeons they did not want to lose their breasts; these surgeons thereupon told them, "You'll be dead within a week if you don't have this mastectomy immediately."

These women became so frightened by the thought of being "dead within a week" that they tearfully submitted to the mastectomies, while they were in a state of a full-blown neurosis.

Some women were told by their surgeons, "You'll be dead tomorrow night if you don't let me do the mastectomy tomorrow morning."

The neurotic woman, who all her life has been afraid to live and is now "scared to death" of dying, accepts this untruth!

One surgeon plays "God" and tells women, "If you let me do the mastectomy tomorrow, I guarantee you that you will live for at least another ten years."

How unconscionable! How dare any surgeon "guarantee" a patient how long she will live! The neurotic woman accepts the word of this "God" and undergoes the radical surgery, whether she needs it or not. Don't let this happen to you!

There are women who, after losing one or perhaps even both of their breasts, say they were never happier in their lives. When people are in very stressful situations and are unable to cope with these situations, they utilize their defense mechanisms.

Defense mechanisms are mental devices which people use to protect their ego against unhappy situations which they are otherwise unable to handle. *Denial* is a popular defense mechanism. This is a disavowal — generally on the unconscious level — of any undesirable feelings, thoughts, needs, deeds or wishes. Thus, the woman who is unhappy about the loss of her breast(s), but cannot cope with this situation, denies the fact that she cries constantly in the confines of her home and says she was never happier than she is now without her breast(s).

There is also a defense mechanism known as *sweet lemon*. This is the reverse of the well known *sour grapes*. Here, the woman rationalizes and says the situation, which she actually finds intolerable (being without one or both of her breasts), is exactly what she has always wanted and that to be without one or both of her breasts is the ideal way to be. — Do you agree? The answer is obvious, isn't it? The women who use the defense mechanisms of *denial* and *sweet lemon* need psychological help.

The MYTH is: If you object to having a mastectomy, you are neurotic.

The FACT is: The woman who has no objection to having a mastectomy is neurotic. The woman who objects has inner emotional strength and self-esteem as a woman and is *not* neurotic.

Myth #4: The woman who has radical surgery demonstrates courage in doing so.
FACT: NO, SHE DOES NOT! It is fear, not courage, that causes her to have radical surgery.

Fear connotes the absence of courage. If the breast cancer patient has courage, she will not permit herself to be readily radically mastectomized.

In all of life's situations, if we are afraid, it is important to admit to ourselves the fact that we are afraid and then to face up to what we fear. Only in this way can we protect ourselves from what we fear. Women who hide their fears and deny their fears are most apt to have radical surgery; they could not admit their fear and, therefore, could not protect themselves against what they feared the most, the radical mastectomy.

When a woman is stricken with a breast disease, terror generally sets in and she thereby becomes vulnerable to excessive surgery. Many a woman who had radical surgery has told me essentially the same story. The story goes as follows:

The woman felt a lump or had a nipple discharge or experienced pain in her breast. She went to her family doctor or her gynecologist, who suggested that she go to the hospital for a "check-up." Arrangements were made for her to be admitted to the hospital and for a surgeon to "examine" her. After she was admitted and was in her hospital bed, a doctor, nurse, nurse's aide or other member of the hospital staff thrust a "consent form" (also known as a "release") at her and told her to sign it.

The hospital atmosphere is often a traumatic one. When she was admitted, the woman was in a state of fright and anxiety about her breasts. The trauma of being in the hospital for possible breast surgery intensified her fear. She was afraid of the member of the hospital staff who thrust the consent form at her. She was not *asked* to sign the release; she was *ordered* to sign it. Nothing was explained to her about the release.

If she hesitated, she was told to hurry up. If she asked a question, she was told she had nothing to worry about and should hurry and sign. In this frightened, traumatized state, she signed the release, quite unaware of the full implications of what she had signed.

She was "prep"ed for surgery, wheeled into the operating room, and put under general anesthesia. Hours later, she awoke in the recovery room and discovered she was minus a breast and that radical surgery had been performed on her. It has taken many women weeks and months and even longer to recover from the shocking discovery that their breasts had been amputated. Some have never recovered.

Don't let his happen to you!

Fear causes a person to lose control over herself. These women had radical surgery because they were overcome by fear. I believe it is a criminal act to put a woman under general anesthesia and amputate her breast without specifically informing her in advance that this would be done to her! Would prison officals dare to amputate a part of a prisoner's body? Of course not! And, of course, they should not! Why are some surgeons doing to innocent women — women who never committed any crime! — what no one would dare to do to even the most hardened criminals!

A release that is signed under duress or when a woman is "non compis mentis" is surely worthless. A woman who is in this state of anxiety and trauma is certainly not fully aware of what she has signed and not mentally capable of responsibly signing a consent form.

Why oh why have these thousands of women so willingly submitted to wanton massive radical breast surgery? Why, in this latter part of the twentieth century, have they not questioned the need for this radical surgery? In a state of self-deception, they have been saying, "See how brave we are," when actually their breast amputations were not at all the result of bravery. They were due to fearfulness, not fearlessness.

The time has come for women to start exhibiting courage by standing up for their rights and their breasts.

The MYTH is: The woman who has radical surgery demonstrates courage in doing so.

The FACT is: It is fear, not courage, that causes her to have radical surgery.

Myth #5: Every breast malignancy requires radical surgery.

FACT: NO, IT DOES NOT! Every breast malignancy does not require radical surgery. With early detection, where the tumor is small and conditions are conducive, lesser surgery and/or radiation therapy may be sufficient and the breast cancer patient's life can be saved and her breast(s) may be spared.

Yes, it is a myth that every breast malignancy requires radical surgery. The radical mastectomy, in which the woman's breast, axillary (armpit) lymph nodes and the pectoral (chest) muscles are removed, has been the most popular mode of treatment for breast cancer in the United States for approximately one hundred years.

In the modified radical mastectomy, the breast plus the axillary lymph nodes are removed, but the chest muscles remain intact. In a simple (sometimes called a "total") mastectomy, only the breast is removed.

In a tylectomy (lumpectomy), the tumor and some healthy surrounding tissue, for safety's sake, are removed and the breast remains intact. There is also a surgical procedure called a "wedge resection." Wedge resection involves the removal of more tissue than in the tylectomy, but the breast is not removed; it is a wider excision, in the form of a wedge, in the area of the tumor. These surgical procedures are known as lesser or conservative surgery in contrast to radical surgery.

The terms "tylectomy," "lumpectomy," "local excision," "conservative surgery" and "lesser surgery" are often used synonymously. Here, as in so many areas of the world of breast cancer, there is controversy. Many physicians agree that these terms are synonymous; some do not. The controversy exists because the amount of tissue removed from the patient's breast may vary with the specific surgical procedure as deemed necessary in each individual case. Some surgeons may remove only the tumor; others may remove varying amounts of tissue in addition to the tumor. In the main, however, the breast remains intact. I am, therefore, using the terms "tylectomy," "lumpectomy," "local excision," "conservative surgery" and "lesser surgery" interchangeably in this book.

After one hundred years and thousands upon thousands of radical mastectomies, the mortality rates for breast cancer patients have not gone down since 1900 (this is as far back as the statistics are available). As a matter of fact, according to some statistics from the National Center for Health Statistics, the mortality rates for breast cancer have been rising.

Each case of breast cancer must be treated on an individual basis. *The treatment should match the individual case.* It should match the malignancy and the host (the patient). Thus, the modern, ethical, competent breast specialist may recommend only radiation therapy (radiation implants or radiation via the external beam) in one case, a tylectomy in another, a wedge resection in a third, a simple mastectomy in a fourth, a modified radical mastectomy in a fifth, and, in a rare case, a radical mastectomy.

Physicians have told me that when Dr. William S. Halsted devised his surgical procedure (the Halsted radical mastectomy) in the nineteenth century, there were no means for early detection of breast cancer. Women's breast tumors were very large when these women presented themselves to their doctors and Dr. Halsted's radical surgery was the only means available then to attempt to save some lives.

We are now in the last quarter of the twentieth century. We now do have means of early detection. Women's breast tumors, when detected, are not the tremendous size they were in the nineteenth century. We now have available better, more effective means of treatment than radical surgery. Yet, although there is a growing trend toward lesser surgery, controversy reigns supreme in the treatment of breast cancer.

When a woman's breast disease is found to be breast cancer, she is in one of the following three situations: 1) her tumor is a local lesion (nodule) in the breast; this is known as "early breast cancer"; 2) the cancer has spread into the axillary (armpit) lymph nodes; or 3) the cancer has spread from the breast to other areas and organs of the body.

There is very little, if any, controversy regarding the treatment when the cancer has spread from the breast to distant areas and organs. Mastectomies are not advised at this stage. The original purpose of the mastectomy was to excise the malignancy and, thereby, hopefully, to prevent its spread to other parts of the body. If this spread has already occurred, a mastectomy is pointless and the patient is generally hospitalized and treated by radiation therapy, chemotherapy, immunotherapy and/or any of the newer therapies which may be coming forth from the cancer research centers and hospitals in the United States and throughout the world.

Most surgeons in the United States are doing radical mastectomies in the stage where the axillary lymph nodes are involved. Some surgeons are doing modified radical mastectomies in such cases. Some breast cancer patients whose lymph nodes are involved refuse mastectomy and permit only the removal of the breast tumor and the involved nodes followed by radiation therapy and/or chemotherapy.

The major controversy rages around "early breast cancer," stage I, for it is where there is a local lesion that a tylectomy and/or radiation therapy can be performed. An increasing number of breast specialists and surgeons are opting for lesser (conservative) surgery and/or radiation therapy in this stage.

The sooner a woman's breast cancer is detected, the greater are the chances of saving her life and also sparing her breast(s). The importance of early detection cannot be overemphasized. With early detection, the malignancy can be caught while it is still a small, local lesion; then, with other conditions conducive, hopefully, the woman's life can be saved and her breast(s) may be spared.

Early detection is based upon MONTHLY BREAST SELF-EXAMINATION and ANNUAL CLINICAL EXAMINATIONS. There is an excellent folder which describes the process of breast self-examination and there is, therefore, no need to describe it here. This folder is called HOW TO EXAMINE YOUR BREASTS and you may obtain a copy free of charge from your local office of the American Cancer Society.

The annual clinical examination should include palpation by the breast specialist and thermography. It should also include mammography if the woman is past the age of fifty or if she is between the ages of thirty-five and fifty and possesses any of the following risk factors: 1) she had cancer in one breast, 2) her mother and/or her sister had pre-menopausal breast cancer, 3) her mother had post-menopausal breast cancer, 4) she has a history of benign breast tumors, or 5) she has lumps in her breast(s), nipple discharge, severe breast pain, or "cystic breasts".

Mammography is a fast, painless procedure in which the breasts are x-rayed. The resulting x-rays are called mammograms. These mammograms enable the breast specialist to determine whether or not there are cancerous tumors within the breast and whether or not any abnormal changes have taken place within the breast. Xerography is a type of mammography which uses a special paper instead of the standard film.

Thermography is also a simple painless procedure and it enables the physician to obtain information about the amount of heat emanating from the breast. This information helps the breast specialist arrive at a judgment about the normal or abnormal state of the woman's breast.

If a woman *does* practice early detection (monthly breast self-examination and annual clinical examinations) and a lump is discovered, and if the lump proves to be malignant, there is good likelihood that the conditions will be conducive to lesser surgery and/or radiation therapy. If a woman *does not* practice early detection and if she has a cancerous tumor, it may grow and spread and she may need the more extensive surgical procedure which she wanted to avoid.

Therefore, I repeat: EARLY DETECTION OF A BREAST CANCER CAN SAVE A WOMAN'S LIFE AND, HOPEFULLY, SPARE HER BREAST(S).

Many women who had radical surgery have told me that as time goes on and they continue to survive, they never cease to worry about metastasis (the spread of the cancer from the original site to other areas and organs of the body). These women worry about metastasis because many of them were told that if they did not have their radical surgery immediately, the cancer cells would spread (metastasize).

So little is known about breast cancer and all cancer that little is known about metastasis too. There are those oncologists (cancer specialists) who believe that by the time a breast tumor is palpable (can be felt by the fingers) or visible, the "seeds" of the cancer have already spread to many other parts of the body. Then, there are those oncologists who say this is not so and that if the tumor is a small, local lesion without any axillary node involvement, there is a good chance that metastasis will never occur if this tumor is removed. There are many oncologists who believe that cancerous cells are present in every human being's body, but there is no malignancy, as such, unless or until millions of these cells group together and form a lump (tumor). Thus, here too controversy reigns supreme.

If a woman's tumor is detected early and it is a small, local lesion and other conditions are conducive, she may be treated by lesser surgery and/or radiation therapy and the likelihood is that metastasis will not occur.

Each breast cancer patient is different. Each case is different. Every cancer is different. There are more than one hundred different cancers. Breast cancer is different from all other cancers and every case of breast cancer is different from every other case. The treatment must be matched with the type of cancer. The mode of treatment must be determined by the total circumstances of each individual case and each individual patient.

The attitude of the modern knowledgeable breast specialist is that he treats a woman and not a cancer. He does not believe that every woman with a malignancy should receive the same treatment. In each case, he matches the treatment to the individual host and her malignancy.

Much depends upon the host and the nature of her cancer. Every host is a different being from every other host. Every breast cancer differs from every other breast cancer in such factors as specific nature of the malignancy, size and location of the tumor, stage of the cancer, rapidity of growth, and the nature of the host (such factors as age, whether premenopausal or postmenopausal, physical condition, emotional state, and the presence of cancer among other members of the family).

Sad to say, breast cancer — like all cancer — is an illness about which little is known, including how to treat it.

Vincent T. DeVita Jr., M.D., Director, Division of Cancer Treatment, National Cancer Institute, U.S. Public Health Service, states, "I believe we don't know how to treat breast cancer at the present time."

Oncologists and physicians of all sorts echo this same sentiment. A noted breast specialist recently said, "We know no more about how to treat breast cancer today than we did forty years ago."

In view of these facts, every effort should be made to spare the woman's breast in addition to saving her life and not to traumatize her by radical surgery. Surely the time has come in this last quarter of the twentieth century to think in terms of lesser surgery, of saving the woman's life and, hopefully, of sparing her breast(s).

For thousands of women who are stricken with breast cancer, it is no longer a choice between their lives and their breasts. With early detection, it is now possible for many of these women to save their lives and their breasts.

Saul Silverman, M.D., Radiation Oncologist at the Radiation Oncology Center of Sutter Community Hospitals in Sacramento, Calif. says, "I think that the vast majority of women with early breast cancer can have effective treatment which preserves the breast."

Let us look at what some other physicians involved with breast cancer say in regard to the treatment of early breast cancer.

M. Vera Peters, M.D., of the Princess Margaret Hospital, Toronto, Ontario, Canada, in her article "Cutting the 'Gordian Knot' in Early Breast Cancer" (ANNALS OF THE ROYAL COLLEGE OF PHYSICIANS AND SURGEONS OF CANADA, July 1975) reports on a 30-year (1939-1969) study of 217 clinical stage I breast cancer patients. These patients were treated by local excision and local radiation. Each of these patients was paired to a patient who was treated by radical or modified radical mastectomy and radiation.

Dr. Peters states, "The quintessence of our profession is that of strengthening the quality of life. Our desire to promote this, coupled with modern detection technology, means no woman in true clinical stage I breast cancer should fall victim to the mental anguish or physical morbidity of radical ways."

She concludes, "This study shows what I have long known to be true; that radical methods are not in the best interest of the patients."

Dr. Peters adds, "Quite apart from the medical disadvantages of mastectomy is the associated emotional trauma, frequently raw and bleeding long after the physical wound becomes a scar. No woman, of any age, contrary to verbal protestations, remains apathetically unresponsive to defeminization — ever the end product of mastectomy!"

Dr. Sakari Mustakallio of the Radiotherapy Clinic, University Central Hospital, Helsinki, Finland, has been using conservative therapy for breast cancer for more than thirty years. In his article, "Conservative Treatment of Breast Carcinoma — Review of 25 Years Follow Up" (CLINICAL RADIOLOGY, THE JOURNAL OF THE ROYAL COLLEGE OF RADIOLOGISTS, 1972, 23, 110-116), he reports on a follow up study of 702 stage I breast cancer patients. By "conservative treatment," Dr. Mustakallio means, "therapy in which the breast is preserved as opposed to radical surgery. The conservative management consists only of local excision of the tumour or of segmental resection and postoperative roentgen therapy." ("Roentgen therapy" is another term for radiation therapy. "Carcinoma" is the technical term for cancer.)

Dr. Mustakallio states, "Conservative treatment of breast carcinoma yields equally good results as any other therapeutic method as regards the patient's life expectancy. Conservative therapy is superior to other methods from the physical and psychic point of view."

He continues, "The classical radical surgery should be abandoned completely in the treatment of mammary carcinoma as it is a harmful method that mutilates the patient."

Knowledgeable oncologists and breast specialists stress that radical surgery traumatizes the patient and trauma prevents the patient from putting up the best possible psychological "fight" against this illness; radical surgery should, therefore, be done only as a last resort. As a psychologist, I am in 100 per cent agreement with this line of thought.

Dr. Mustakallio likewise states, "As a patient's own powers of resistance to tumour growth are very important for her life expectancy, traumatisation of the patient should be avoided as far as possible."

He concludes, "I believe that only when we change our local line of thinking and treatment, so common in cancer research, to a more dynamic approach that takes into account the whole organism of the cancer patient and examine and treat the patient accordingly, can we expect an appreciable reduction in the mortality rate of mammary carcinoma."

In his article, "Treatment of Early Breast Cancer," (BULLETIN OF THE MASON CLINIC, Spring 1975), Dr. John L. Hayward, Fellow of the Royal College of Surgeons, Director, Breast Unit, Guy's Hospital, London, England, concludes with a consideration of why many women are not interested in going to screening centers for the detection of early breast cancer.

Dr. Hawyard states, "They are not interested for two reasons. One, they are frightened of getting cancer and there is not much we can do about this except to continue public education. The second thing they are frightened of is a mutilating operation. Each one is frightened that if somebody finds she has a carcinoma, she will lose her breast. If we can just hint to these people that if we get the tumor at its earliest stage, a mutilating operation may not be necessary, it is my belief that they will come earlier. And so with conservative surgery for early disease, we may have something life-saving to offer."

Alfred C. Meyer, M.D. and Simmons S. Smith, M.D. present an analysis of 1,686 surgically treated carcinomas of the breast in their article, "Carcinoma of the Breast: A Clinical Study" (ARCHIVES OF SURGERY, April 1978). In conclusion, they state, "Radical mastectomy does not increase survival compared to more conservative operations and should therefore be abandoned except in special circumstances."

In early breast cancer, the breast can be spared not only by conservative surgery, but also by solely radiation therapy. Reports of this type of treatment for breast carcinoma have appeared in medical journals for the past two decades, but until recently the American medical profession has paid little attention to them.

Leonard R. Prosnitz, M.D. and Ira S. Goldenberg, M.D. of Yale University School of Medicine and Yale-New Haven Hospital, New Haven, Connecticut, describe a treatment program for early stage breast cancer in their article, "Radiation Therapy as Primary Treatment for Early Stage Carcinoma of the Breast" (CANCER, June 1975). The treatment plan in this program consisted of biopsy only and primary radiation therapy.

"To preserve the breast and avoid the mutilation of mastectomy" were the objectives of this treatment program.

Dr. Prosnitz and Dr. Goldenberg conclude, "Much suggestive evidence has now accumulated that primary radiation therapy is as effective as mastectomy in the management of early stage breast carcinoma. Possibly it is more effective. Such treatment must be carried out with a full understanding of the radio-biological principles involved if optimum results are to be achieved."

They add, "Finally, it has been suggested that if primary radiation therapy without mastectomy is as effective a method of treatment as mastectomy and the fear of losing a breast is lessened, more women may seek attention earlier for breast lumps, with a resultant increase in survival."

At the Harvard Medical School, Department of Radiation Therapy, Joint Center for Radiation Therapy in Boston, 150 patients with localized breast cancer were treated by radiation therapy without mastectomy in the period between July 1, 1968 and December 31, 1974. In their article, "Treatment of Carcinoma of the Breast by Radiation Therapy" (CANCER, June 1977), Martin B. Levene, M.D., Jay R. Harris, M.D. and Samuel Hellman, M.D. present their results with these patients. They state, "Radiation therapy without mastectomy is a local treatment which offers the potential for local control with minimal functional or cosmetic impairment."

They conclude, "Our results to date suggest that radiation therapy following gross excision of the primary tumor is a highly effective means of achieving local control in cancer of the breast. Thus far there have been no local failures in any of the Stage I or II patients."

I want to keep this book within attractively readable size and, therefore, I do not wish, nor do I think it necessary, to discuss here any additional studies showing the advantages of conservative surgery and/or radiation therapy over that of radical surgery in the treatment of early breast cancer. The treatment of breast cancer is changing rapidly and surely the time is not far off when radical surgery will be abandoned as a mode of treatment of breast cancer.

The MYTH is: Every breast malignancy requires radical surgery.

The FACT is: Every breast malignancy does not require radical surgery. With early detection, where the tumor is small and conditions are conducive, lesser surgery and/or radiation therapy may be sufficient and the breast cancer patient's life can be saved and her breast(s) may be spared.

Part Two

From
Tumor
To
Verdict
To
Choice

PART II

FROM TUMOR TO VERDICT TO CHOICE

I am enough of a baseball fan to have heard of the expression "from Tinker to Evers to Chance." When Tinker skillfully threw the ball to Evers who then threw it to Chance, it was a double play, two men were "out," and the game was won.

In the "game" of life, thousands upon thousands of people annually are faced with "from tumor to verdict to choice." "Winning" here depends to a great extent upon the breast specialists, surgeons and other physicians, and additionally, upon each patient's mind, upon the psychological constitution and emotional strength of the individual patient.

Much depends upon the patient's possession of a positive attitude, a positive outlook, and the definite determination to live — and, not just to live, but to live effectively.

Every year more than a million women become aware that there is trouble brewing in their breasts. Some have "shooting pains" through their nipple(s) and/or nipple discharges. Others feel pain throughout one or both of their breasts. Still others discover, by means of mammography or by breast self-examination, what could best be termed "terrifying tumors," for a tumor in a woman's breast is surely terrifying to her. Yet others become aware of a miscellany of other breast abnormalities. These abnormal conditions are symptomatic of any one of a variety of breast diseases.

What should a woman do when she becomes aware of the fact that she has a breast disease?

She should go immediately to her family physician, who should recommend to her a breast specialist who knows all there is to know about breast diseases. You can give yourself the maximum advantage by going to a specialist who is most knowledgeable about breast diseases, who knows everything that is known to the medical profession about breast diseases, benign (non-cancerous) as well as malignant (cancerous).

Unfortunately, the American medical profession does not have a specific medical specialty concerned with diseases and disorders of the breast. There should be such a specialty, just as there are specialties concerned with other organs of the body, such as cardiology which is concerned with diseases and disorders of the heart.

At present, it is the radiologist who comes closest to being the "breast specialist" and this is the physician to whom I am referring when I speak of the "breast specialist" in this book. This is the physician, the medical specialist, to whom the woman should go. She should not go directly to a surgeon for if she does, she has chosen her mode of treatment before knowing whether surgery should be the mode of treatment in her particular case. The radiologist specializes in the diagnosis and treatment of diseases and disorders of the human body by means of x-rays and radioactive substances. The radiologist who further specializes in the diagnosis and treatment of illnesses of the breast is known as a breast specialist or breast diagnostician.

31

The woman should be honest with herself. She should not fool herself. She has too much at stake. Her life and her breasts are at stake. There are women who insist they know "everything" about breast cancer. I have found that these are the women who know the least about this illness. If they knew "anything" about breast cancer, they would know that even the most knowledgeable specialists do not know "everything" about breast cancer. Unfortunately, so little about breast cancer — or any other cancer — is known even to the medical profession. Certainly, the average person could not be expected to know very much about this illness. So, no woman should feel ashamed of not knowing much about breast cancer.

Those women who fool themselves into thinking they know a lot about their breasts when in reality they know very little are most apt to become victims of excessive surgery.

It is shocking that even the basic known facts about this illness are so unknown to most women. Not only are most American women so very uninformed about their breasts and breast diseases, but they are also woefully misinformed on this subject. I was surprised recently to hear a woman college graduate, with a Phi Beta Kappa key dangling from her neck, speak of a "massectomy." There is no such thing as a "massectomy." The term is "mastectomy."

The woman who has been stricken with a benign breast disease, such as a benign breast tumor, should certainly go to a breast specialist for annual clinical examinations, in addition to practicing monthly breast self-examination, for she is more vulnerable to breast cancer than women who have not been stricken with a benign breast disease.

If a woman has a breast tumor and she goes to a competent, knowledgeable breast specialist, if her tumor proves to be malignant — and, if she has been practicing the rules of early detection and immediate consultation with a breast specialist — her chances of being cured of breast cancer are enhanced and she will be unlikely to become a victim of excessive surgery.

Women must become "partners" with their breast specialists in the care and treatment of their breasts. The cause(s) of breast cancer is unknown. Until the cause is discovered, the best protection is to practice monthly breast self-examination and to go to a breast specialist for annual clinical examinations.

If a tumor is detected, the likelihood is that the tumor is benign, since approximately seven to eight out of ten tumors of the breast are benign. Often the breast specialist can determine from his examinations whether or not the tumor is malignant. However, the physician may want the patient to go to the hospital for a biopsy of the tumor.

A biopsy is a limited surgical procedure in which the entire tumor (if the tumor is small) or a small amount of tissue from the tumor (if the tumor is large) is removed for microscopic examination to determine whether the tumor is benign or malignant.

If you go to a hospital for a biopsy, you have the right to decide whether or not to sign the hospital consent form (release). If you decide to sign the release, be sure it specifically states that you are granting permission for a biopsy — and only a biopsy — to be performed. Biopsies are performed under local anesthesia.

The release form should be presented to the patient before she is admitted to the hospital and she should be permitted to read it — all of it, including the "small print" — at home in as relaxed a state as possible. She should have the right to decide whether or not she wishes to sign it as it is or whether she would like to make some changes in it. Only she, the patient, should have the right to sign the release — not her husband or other relative or anyone else! The ultimate decision should rest with her — it is her life, her body and her breast(s)!

Traditionalist surgeons believe that if the biopsy indicates the tumor is malignant, radical surgery should be performed immediately. They want the patient to sign the consent form giving them the right to do as they see fit. They then perform the biopsy while the patient is under general anesthesia. If the biopsy proves to be positive, these surgeons proceed to perform radical surgery. This is known as the "one-step" procedure.

Thus, if the woman does not stipulate on the release that she is granting permission for a biopsy only, she will be put under general anesthesia and she may awake to the shock of discovering that her breast was removed while she thought she had gone into the hospital for a biopsy only.

Some women want to know the results of the biopsy before anything further is done to them. If their biopsy proves to be positive, they want time to consider their options. This is known as the "two-step" procedure in contrast to the "one-step" procedure. In the "two-step" procedure, there is a time interval between the biopsy and further surgery.

On the basis of the many discussions I have had with numerous physicians, I believe I am justified in saying that there is no risk in a short delay between the biopsy and any further surgery. This interval between the biopsy and further treatment gives the patient the opportunity to consider the options (alternative modes of treatment) available to her. She needs the time to discuss the matter with her breast specialist, her surgeon, her family physician, her family, her friends, and/or others with whom she may wish to consult. If her surgeon insists on a radical mastectomy — or, for that matter, any other mastectomy — she may wish to go to another surgeon for consultation. After all of this consultation, the patient should digest the results, do a lot of thinking, and come to her own decision of her own free will — for the ultimate decision should rest with her.

There are some women who may prefer the "one-step" procedure. They state that if the biopsy is positive the surgeon has their permission to perform a mastectomy on them. Thus, many of these women make their "choice" without ever hearing the "it's malignant" verdict. These women do not want any time interval between their biopsy and further surgery, if further surgery is deemed necessary. This is their right.

I want women to know that "one-step" and "two-step" procedures are available to them and they have the right to choose which of these procedures they prefer. What they do with the hospital consent form will depend upon whether they choose the "one-step" or the "two-step" procedure.

Some women may also wish to discuss the subject of anesthesia with their surgeons. Breast biopsies may be performed under local anesthesia. These biopsies may be performed in ambulatory surgical units, often in the smaller operating rooms in the OPD (Out-Patient Department) rather than in the main operating rooms of large hospitals. One-day surgery is becoming increasingly popular for certain surgical procedures, such as breast biopsies and other lesser surgical procedures, in many hospitals throughout the country. Local anesthesia is sufficient under such circumstances. General anesthesia has its hazards and is not necessary for breast biopsies.

Those women who are told their tumors are benign should thank God for it and heave a sigh of relief. For them, it is "from tumor to verdict."

What if the woman is told her tumor is malignant? Two to three out of every ten breast tumors prove to be cancerous. For these women, the verdict is, "it's malignant." For them, it now becomes, "from tumor to verdict to choice."

The woman who is told she has breast cancer is faced with the most difficult dilemma of her life. She has received the verdict. Now, she must make the choice, essentially the choice between lesser surgery and radical surgery for even if she were to choose radiation therapy only, the tumor is often surgically removed first. This choice is an extremely difficult one.

Since most women are, unfortunately, uninformed and misinformed about their breasts and breast diseases, on what basis can they possibly make a rational choice in so vital a matter?

There are two bases for choice. One is the medical basis. The other is the psychological basis.

For the medical basis, the woman must primarily depend upon her physician. She must trust and have faith in her physician. If she does not trust him (or her) or have faith in him (or her), she should get another physician. Here, too, a woman should be careful not to fool herself. Most general practitioners, internists, family physicians, and all other physicians other than breast specialists, unfortunately, know little about breast cancer. Unless the woman is in the care of a knowledgeable breast specialist, she is in all likelihood in the care of a physician who knows little about breast diseases, benign as well as malignant.

The knowledgeable breast specialist may offer the breast cancer patient his recommendation for the mode of treatment in her case or he may offer her options (alternative modes of treatment) from among which she may make her choice.

However, essentially, it is the woman's mind, her psychological constitution, that will determine her mode of treatment.

Your mind — your psychological constitution — will largely determine whether you will choose lesser surgery or radical surgery, if you are faced with this choice. How you feel toward yourself, toward others, and toward the totality of your past and present environments and experiences will influence this vital decision.

Answer the following nine questions with a "Yes" or "No":
1. Are you afraid of death?
2. Do you have faith in God?
3. Do you have a strong feeling of self-esteem as a woman?
4. Do you feel needed and wanted by family and friends?
5. Are you a non-conformist, unafraid to leave the mainstream?
6. Are you negatively inclined toward surgery, surgery of any kind?
7. Do you feel young?
8. Is cancer rare in your family?
9. Do you have a positive mental outlook toward life?

If the majority of your replies are, "Yes," you will tend to opt for lesser surgery. If the majority of your replies are, "No," you will tend to opt for radical surgery.

Unquestionably, some of these questions carry more weight with some women than with others. However, these questions are not the result of a scientific survey and there is, therefore, no basis upon which to give each question a specific "point" weight. They are the fruits of my experience in intensively and extensively investigating the world of breast cancer since I was stricken with breast cancer in July 1975.

Some of these questions are more emotionally charged than others and her response to any one of the emotionally charged questions may tend to veer a woman toward either lesser surgery or radical surgery, regardless of her responses to the other questions. Thus, a majority of "Yes"'s or "No"'s may not be necessary if a woman feels particularly sensitive or responsive to one specific question; her response to that one question may determine her choice of treatment.

There is one question that I would like to single out for special consideration and that is question #8. The genetic factor in breast cancer is a biological factor. However, how we react to this factor depends upon our psychological constitution. If a woman belongs to a family in which breast cancer appears to "run" in the family, this factor alone will carry tremendous weight in her choice of treatment if she is stricken with breast cancer. The breast cancer patient who has a premenopausal mother and other relatives who were stricken with breast cancer is surely more likely to choose radical surgery than lesser surgery and cannot be faulted for doing so.

As you read and review the other eight questions, there may be those of you who will say unhappily, "More than a majority of my replies are 'No,' so that means I am doomed to radical surgery if I get breast cancer."

It doesn't mean anything of the kind. You are not at all "doomed to radical surgery." We are none of us "doomed" to anything. We can change our psychological constitution. You may say that you can't change. That is not so. *You can change if you want to change.*

With every single question, except #8, (the aforementioned genetic factor), change is possible. In some instances, you can accomplish this change yourself; in other instances, psychological counseling may be necessary.

Let us examine each of these questions.

1. Are you afraid of death?

This I have already discussed in Part I, Myth #1. Let me add here that I believe it is extremely important to break the chain of thinking that links together "death" and "breast cancer" in the minds of some people. Breast cancer, as I said in Part I, is *not* a death sentence.

Those who are afraid of death should give some deep thought to this question. This is very important for the more afraid you are of death, the more likely you are to choose radical surgery.

Ask yourself: what is death? It is the shedding of one's earthly clothing. That's all that your body is — earthly clothing to house your mind and your soul. Your soul continues on after death. So, if you are afraid of death — what is it that you are afraid of?

Children are afraid of death and justifiably so. You are not a child. The woman who is afraid of death has not grown up and is still a child; she has become fixated at the pre-adolescent, little girl stage. This "little girl woman", so afraid of death and so accepting of myths, if she is stricken with breast cancer, will, due to fear, probably opt for radical surgery. The mature woman, unafraid of death and unaccepting of myths, if she is stricken with breast cancer, will probably opt for lesser surgery.

A woman who had a radical mastectomy said to me recently, "I could have had a lumpectomy, but I was afraid I might die." This woman prides herself on her knowledge of medicine and science, yet her knowledge of these subjects had nothing to do with her choice of radical surgery. Her choice was based upon the fact that she "was afraid I might die" — and the fact that she was prodded toward radical surgery by a traditionalist surgeon. She admitted that her knowledge caused her to question the value of radical surgery in her case, but fear overwhelmed her.

2. Do you have faith in God?

If you have faith in God, you will tend to believe in the Biblical dictum, "Thy will be done." If you have faith in God, you will also tend to believe that you remain on this earth as long as the good Lord so wishes and only He knows how long you will remain here.

The medical profession admits that there are many, many unanswered questions regarding breast cancer. The medical profession does not know what is the best treatment for breast cancer. In such a situation, even if you have the highest regard for the medical profession, as I do, if you have faith in God, you will tend to choose lesser surgery.

It is important to differentiate here between true faith in God and pseudo-religion. The truly religious person adheres to the Golden Rule; do unto others as you want others to do unto you. The person who has true faith in God reveres God and marvels at His accomplishments. This person, depending upon personal circumstances, may or may not practice certain traditions of her religion.

The pseudo-religious person is one who practices many, perhaps all, of the traditions of her religion, but does not practice the Golden Rule. This pseudo-religious woman tries to give others the impression that she is religious, when, in fact, she is not. She does not revere God; she fears God. This fear, plus all the other fears that motivate such a woman, will tend to veer her toward radical surgery.

Thus, the woman who reveres God is apt to opt for lesser surgery; the woman who fears God is apt to opt for radical surgery.

3. Do you have a strong feeling of self-esteem as a woman?

This has little, if anything, to do with whether a woman is married or single. There are thousands upon thousands of women who have been married for ten, twenty, thirty or even more years, who have very little self-esteem as a woman and who are very insecure in their feminine sexuality. It has a great deal to do with whether you feel that men are attracted to you and have respect for you.

The woman who has a strong feeling of self-esteem as a woman will tend toward lesser surgery; the woman who has little feeling of self-esteem as a woman will tend toward radical surgery.

If you do not have a strong feeling of self-esteem as a woman, psychological counseling would be advisable to get to the roots of why you feel as you do; change could not be achieved unless you understand why you feel inadequate and insecure. Perhaps some years ago, you were rejected by the one man you wanted and you have carried your past into your present, despite the fact that you may be married for a number of years to the man you married on the rebound. Perhaps at present, you are married to a man who is unresponsive to you. There are a multitude of reasons which may cause you to feel as you do and psychological counseling could be of help to you.

I would like to mention here the subject of "breast mystique." It is true that the breast is a very emotionally charged organ. It is true too that every normal woman wants to protect and keep her breasts. Although the advertising world certainly has played up the breast as a sex symbol, the mature, well adjusted woman's feeling of self-esteem as a woman is based not solely on her breast(s), but on her total being. However, this does not mean that this woman is willing to part with her breast(s). Loss of her breast(s) is defeminizing and no normal woman wants to be defeminized.

The mature, well-adjusted woman with her strong feeling of self-esteem as a woman has an accompanying strong feeling of self-worth and is, therefore, unafraid to ask questions. She may question whether it is truly necessary for her breast(s) to be amputated in view of the fact that the medical profession does not know what is the best treatment for breast cancer; she may question why she should suffer the subsequent trauma and pain, particularly since there is no evidence that chances of survival are increased. She may ask ever so many questions and then she will probably tend toward lesser surgery.

4. Do you feel needed and wanted by family and friends?

To feel needed and wanted means to feel loved. To feel loved means to feel somebody cares. To love someone means to care for that person. Love may range in intensity from simple affection to the deepest devotion of a woman for a man and vice versa. There are many different kinds of love. There is not just the love of woman for man and man for woman, there is love for one's children, parents, grandparents, siblings and other relatives, and friends.

The more needed and wanted you feel, the more confident you are that there are people who love you and care about what happens to you, and the greater is your feeling of inner security. The greater this feeling, the more apt you are to choose lesser surgery. The woman who feels uneeded, unwanted, unloved is more apt to choose radical surgery.

Many women have no close friends and find it difficult to form friendships. If you have no close friends, ask yourself to whom you are a friend. You must first be a friend before you can have a friend. You may be too self-involved and not sufficiently other-involved. You must make efforts in this direction. It may be possible for you yourself to make the necessary changes in your psychological constitution to enable you to achieve close friendships. If you find this difficult to do, then you may need psychological counseling.

5. Are you a nonconformist, unafraid to leave the mainstream?

If you are a nonconformist, you take risks and are unafraid of failure. Criticism does not deter you. You agree with that famous expression: "To avoid criticism, do nothing, say nothing, be nothing," and you believe in doing something, saying something, and being something.

Nonconformists are unafraid to go out and "fight" for what they want and for what they believe to be true. They take chances and accept challenges and, thereby, live an outwardly insecure, non-sheltered existence, but inwardly they feel quite secure.

When I received my doctor's degree, I decided to leave a "secure," well-paying position to go into private practice and become self-employed. Many people said to me, "Don't do it. Don't take chances." They were trying to foist their insecurities onto me. I did not let them. I took chances and have never regretted doing so; life has been ever so much more meaningful and exciting as a result of the chances I took and the challenges I accepted.

Life has many problems. If you are a nonconformist, there are additional problems; but, you are an independent person and can "take it" for you have what is known as "high frustration tolerance."

If you are a conformist, you are a dependent person, generally afraid to take risks, afraid of criticism, afraid of failure. You have been living a rather sheltered, "cocoon-like" existence. Everything around you appears secure, such as "secure" home, "secure" job, "secure" pension, but inwardly you are very insecure.

The conformist who has had a rather easy, comfortable, financially secure life has not had the opportunity to develop any "frustration tolerance." Due to "low frustation tolerance," this person finds problems hard to take and simply can't "take it."

The nonconformist, unafraid to leave the mainstream, is apt to opt for lesser surgery. The conformist can't "take it" and is, therefore, apt to opt for radical surgery, the popular "mainstream" mode of treatment for breast cancer. If you would like to raise your frustration tolerance, professional psychological help is advisable; group guidance sessions would be especially helpful for this purpose.

6. Are you negatively inclined toward surgery, surgery of any kind?

The person who readily obeys authority and docilely takes orders from all authority figures, including her physician, is generally positively inclined toward surgery. This person does not question "why." Her surgeon says she needs surgery; therefore, she will have surgery performed on her. This woman will choose radical surgery.

I admit that I am very negatively inclined toward surgery, surgery of any kind. I feel this way as a result of the totality of my life's experiences with persons for whom I have cared, persons close to me. The only surgery I ever had, other than my "lesser breast surgery," was the removal of my tonsils and adenoids when I was very young. This was popular when I was a little girl and my parents certainly meant well when they had this done. However, I am sorry it was done. Tonsils and adenoids are filters and I believe that if I still had my tonsils and adenoids, I, living in highly polluted New York City, would have less trouble with my sinuses than I have.

I want to emphasize here that I have the greatest respect for my surgeon. He is an excellent surgeon and has performed superb surgery on me. I also readily give credit to the members of the surgical profession for the countless thousands upon thousands of lives they have saved and the many recent "miracles" they have performed. However, as for myself, personally, I would never permit any amputation of any part of my body to be performed on me, and, I pray, the good Lord willing, that no such surgery will ever be deemed necessary. If I believed it were necessary, I would agree to lesser surgery.

The woman who is negatively inclined toward surgery does not docilely take orders from authority figures. She questions "why." This woman tends toward lesser surgery. The woman who is positively inclined toward surgery tends toward radical surgery.

7. Do you feel young?

This question is not: "Are you young?" It is: "Do you *feel* young?

I am asking about your psychological age, rather than your chronological age. Your psychological age is the determinant here and not your chronological age.

The psychologically young person may be in her fifties or her seventies or even in her nineties, but she looks forward toward the future with zest and enthusiasm. The psychologically old person may be in her twenties or thirties, but she dwells more in the past than in the present and does not look forward to the future. The psychologically young woman looks forward; the psychologically old woman looks backward.

The woman who feels young, who looks forward to the future is apt to opt for lesser surgery. The woman who feels old, who looks backward to the past, is apt to opt for radical surgery.

8. Is cancer rare in your family?

Earlier, I singled out this question for special consideration. I stated that the breast cancer patient whose mother and other relatives had breast cancer is more likely to choose radical surgery and should not be faulted for doing so.

Interestingly, however, some women whose mothers were stricken with breast cancer have told me that they are very conscientiously practicing early detection; if they are stricken with breast cancer, it will be detected at an early stage and, they say, they may consider lesser surgery. Thus, depending upon the psychological constitution of the individual woman, lesser surgery may be a possibility here too.

If breast cancer is rare in the breast cancer patient's family, especially if neither her mother nor any other close relative had breast cancer, she may tend to give consideration to lesser surgery.

9. Do you have a positive mental outlook toward life?

If you do not have a positive mental outlook, you feel your situation is quite hopeless. You are a pessimist and feel that tomorrow will be even worse than today. You are a worrier and often feel depressed.

If you have a positive mental outlook, you are full of hope and optimism. You are rarely depressed and, when you do feel depressed, it is of short duration. You believe "the wheel turns" and tomorrow will be better. You waste little time at worrying for life is too precious to waste. No matter how tough the troubles, you try to maintain a cheerful attitude for you agree with the Bible's "a merry heart doeth good like a medicine."

There are people who more or less make up their minds that they will not get well, that they will get sicker; the chances are that these people will not get well and will get sicker. There are those who make up their minds that they will get well; the chances are great that they will get well. This is known as the self-fulfilling prophecy.

Thus, if you have a positive mental outlook, the likelihood is that you will choose lesser surgery. If you have a negative mental outlook, the likelihood is that you will choose radical surgery. If you are depressed and are overcome by a negative mental outlook, psychological counseling should prove to be of much value to you.

If you find yourself with a majority of "No" replies to these nine questions and are not pleased about this, get to work at changing your psychological constitution. Remember, you can change if you really want to change. You may need professional help to accomplish this change. If you do, there are many certified psychologists who are qualified to help you.

Go to your local public library and ask the librarian for a copy of the book entitled NATIONAL REGISTER OF HEALTH SERVICE PROVIDERS IN PSYCHOLOGY. In this book, you will be able to locate qualified psychologists who have satisfied all requirements as to training and experience necessary for them to receive a certificate and to be recognized by the Council for the National Register of Health Service Providers in Psychology as a health service provider in psychology. They are listed geographically and this will help you locate a qualified psychologist who practices near your home.

So, it is you — the individual woman — who decides on your mode of treatment if you are stricken with a malignancy and you choose on the basis of your mind, your psychological constitution.

Your mind makes the choice. Your mind can fight breast cancer: 1) by choosing your mode of treatment, and 2) by generating the positive attitudes and the overall positive mental outlook needed to overcome the onslaught of the cancerous cells.

Your mind can generate the healthy will to live — the inner determination and positive attitudes — to get well and stay well. Let your mind do it. Don't hinder it; help it. Your mind has a difficult task in the fight against breast cancer. It needs all the help it can get.

Now, perhaps you would like to know how one woman went FROM TUMOR TO VERDICT TO CHOICE. Read on and you will learn about what I did.

Experiences - Personal and Personnel

EXPERIENCES — PERSONAL AND PERSONNEL

Cancer is a mugger. It creeps up on you stealthily and often tries to kill you; too often it succeeds. The mugger is a social cancer. He also creeps up on you stealthily and often tries to kill you; too often he too succeeds.

In the summer of '75, I was determined to conquer the external mugger, the social cancer, as well as the internal mugger, the physiological cancer.

Police often say that people who are mugged are generally not in a state of 100 per cent alertness. I certainly was not 100 per cent alert that day in September 1975 when I left my favorite department store and walked down Third Avenue.

Since July 18, 1975, when I heard the dreaded words, "it's malignant," I had been talking with many physicians about the detection, prevention and treatment of breast cancer. Now, I was preparing to fly to visit my very wonderful, warm-hearted friends, Eve and Al Chaiken, at whose house I would stay while keeping appointments with doctors at the prestigious Samson Cancer Center. I had to do some necessary shopping in preparation for this trip.

It was a beautiful, sunny September day and I was deep in thought as I strolled along Third Avenue in a leisurely manner, contrary to my usual quick walk. It is not easy to be deep in thought on New York City's Third Avenue, with all of the noise of the heavy traffic, construction, and pot-hole drilling. However, as a native New Yorker, I have learned not only to ignore this noise, but to be totally oblivious to it.

Suddenly, I felt something sharp jabbing at my back and I heard the mugger's whispered words, "Gimme your money."

Without a moment's hesitation, I swirled around, swung my purse straight at his stomach and lustily said, "I had a cancer operation. I'm not afraid of cancer and I'm not afraid of you."

I had taken him by surprise. The mugger froze at my gaze and my words. He was a youngster of no more than fourteen or fifteen years of age. We stared at each other for a few seconds. His eyes were shining with a combination of shock, sadness and sympathy. He stood still as though paralyzed or in a trance and mumbled, "Geez, cancer."

"Yes, cancer," I said. "I won't let cancer kill me. And I won't let you kill me either."

"Geez, I'm sorry." He paused and repeated, "Geez, I'm sorry you have cancer."

The expression of sympathy had spread across his face. I could not help but think what a strange world this is. Here was a young mugger evincing sympathy. This was September 11th. I thought back to the July day when I consulted Dr. Pheless, the "well known breast surgeon" at the "well known medical center" — this surgeon with his repulsive, snarling face who had not one word of compassion, who never said even as much as a "good-bye and good luck." The mugger was more human — more humane — than that surgeon.

I asked the young mugger to give me his knife. He swore he did not have one. His hands were empty. I had turned around so fast that had he had a knife or any other weapon, it would still have been in his hand. He turned his pockets inside out to prove to me that he had no weapon of any kind on him. He said he had poked his finger into my back.

"O.K. then, let's go for a walk down Third Avenue," I ordered.

I started to walk. He followed obediently. We continued in the direction I had been walking. I told him that I am a counseling psychologist, that I had been a school counselor, that I had counseled thousands of young and older people, and that I would like to help him.

As we walked down the avenue, we discussed his schooling. He said his high school was closed because the teachers were on strike. He tried to use the strike as justification for his mugging and swore that this was his first attempt at mugging someone. I told him there is no excuse, no justification for mugging.

We continued walking and talking. We discussed the subjects he was studying, his likes and dislikes, the courses in which he excelled, and the special interests and aptitudes he possessed. During our stroll, he had come to trust me and so he was talking in a very relaxed manner. This twelve-block stroll is probably the most unique counseling session I have ever conducted.

Suddenly, he stopped talking and stood still. Fear had swept across his face. I wondered what had happened. And, then I knew.

We had reached 42nd Street. There was a traffic cop at the intersection of 42nd Street and Third Avenue. This was the first police officer we had encountered along the way.

He was frightened. "You gonna have me arrested?"

"Of course not," I said quickly.

He believed me and he relaxed.

"I'm not interested in having you arrested. I am interested in helping you to become a decent, law-abiding citizen," I said.

I suggested that we step into the cafeteria on the corner of 42nd and Third to have a bite and to continue our conversation. He came along hesitantly. We crossed the street, passed the traffic cop, and entered the restaurant. I suspected he was hesitant because he had no money — and I was correct. I told him to buy the food he liked and I would pay for it.

After we made our purchases, we carried our trays to a table. I did not ask him his name or the name of the high school he attended so he would not have the slightest fear that I would report his aborted mugging.

We ate and chatted about his future. I was impressed with his articulateness and intelligence. We discussed colleges and the careers he might someday enter. I told him of the financial aid he could get to help him go to college. We also discussed a problem that was bothering him and I hope I helped him to cope with it.

Forty-five minutes had passed. We finished eating and I had to be on my way to an appointment. As we went through the revolving door and out of the cafeteria, he promised me that he would never again attempt to mug anyone. I said the teachers' strike would be over and the schools would probably re-open on Monday. I suggested that he see his school counselor about a program change he wanted and about his future career plans.

As we shook hands in parting, I handed him a few dollar bills. I wanted him to have some money for the coming weekend. He refused to take them.

"You paid for my meal. I can't take anymore money from you" he hesitated and then added — "you have cancer, you need the money."

I did not want to bring up the fact that just about an hour earlier, he had wanted to take the money from me illegally. I simply said, "That's all right. I want you to buy something, go to a movie, or do whatever you wish with it to enjoy the weekend."

I insisted that he take the money. This time, he took it. He thanked me profusely and said, "I'm gonna pray for you. I'm gonna pray that you shouldn't have cancer."

He stopped for a moment. He was overcome with emotion. Then, he added, "I'm gonna pray that you should be healthy and that you should live for a real long time."

I thanked him. We wished each other good health and good luck and we parted. I am hopeful that this boy will be all right, that someday he will be a self-supporting, self-respecting, law-abiding citizen.

Let us go back a few months preceding this mugging episode. I had ben discomforted for several months due to what my family physician had called, "cystic mastitis," a benign breast disease; no lump was present. Then, one day, my family physician, Dr. Legume, and I were able to feel a tiny tumor.

I am fortunate that Dr. Legume referred me to Dr. Knowals, the foremost breast specialist. On June 10, 1975, I was in Dr. Knowals' offices where mammography, thermography and clinical examinations were conducted. On the basis of the test results and certain symptoms, there was reason to hope that the tumor might be benign.

I shall not describe the symptoms here because if I do, some women might be tempted to do self-diagnosis of a breast condition of their own. SELF-EXAMINATION of your breasts is very important. SELF-DIAGNOSIS is very dangerous. There are competent, breast specialists and only they, not you, should diagnose the condition of your breasts.

Dr. Knowals showed me the mammograms (breast x-rays) and explained to me why there was basis to believe that the tiny tumor in my breast was a papilloma (a benign tumor arising from a papilla). He asked me a number of questions including some on my family history. I told him there had never been any breast cancer or any other cancer in my family as far back as my great grandparents.

Although there was a 90 per cent likelihood that the tumor was a papilloma, there was still that ten per cent of doubt. Dr. Knowals said, "Since what you have in your breast is a foreign body, I would like to be on the safe side and have it removed."

He added that the medical profession does not know when a lump — papilloma or any other kind — might be a cancer and, therefore, it would be best to remove it.

The prospect of surgery did not please me. However, I was very impressed with Dr. Knowals and what he said made sense. Unfortunately, the medical profession knows neither what causes, nor how to prevent, nor what is the best mode of treatment of breast cancer. But, I do believe that Dr. Knowals knows all there is to know — and more. He is a very compassionate man, truly concerned about the health of his patients. So, although I am quite anti-surgery, I agreed to undergo this surgery for the removal of the little lump.

Before referring me back to Dr. Legume who would make the hospital arrangements, Dr. Knowals told me that the surgery I would undergo would take from fifteen to twenty minutes. Then, he advised me to follow these stipulations: 1) the surgery to remove the tumor should be done under local anesthesia and not general anesthesia, 2) it should be done in the small operating room in the outpatient department (OPD) and not in the hospital's main operating room, and,

3) I should not sign a hospital release giving the hospital and the surgeon permission to do whatever they please.

After receiving the report from Dr. Knowals, Dr. Legume made arrangements at Tenderloin, a well-known "teaching" hospital. The surgeon at Tenderloin agreed to all of Dr. Knowals' stipulations. I was scheduled to go in for surgery, Tuesday, July 1st, 1975.

I was told the surgeon's name was Dr. Shautt. Before you permit a surgeon to operate on you, you should check on his credentials. I checked on Dr. Shautt in the DIRECTORY OF MEDICAL SPECIALISTS and found that he is a board certified surgeon. Dr. Legume also told me that Dr. Shautt is known to be a capable surgeon.

I asked other physicians too about Dr. Shautt and they also said he is competent. However, I discovered some time ago, and now found it to be true again, that one physician's view of a second physician is quite often at variance with a patient's view of the second physician. The physician is concerned about whether the surgeon has capable hands; the patient wants the surgeon to have capable hands and, equally and probably even more important, a compassionate heart.

On Thursday, June 26th, I received a phone call from Dr. Legume telling me that Dr. Shautt had changed his mind and was now insisting that my surgery should be performed in the main operating room under general anesthesia. Under no circumstances would I permit this.

Dr. Legume suggested that I phone Dr. Shautt and discuss the matter with him. I phoned Dr. Shautt immediately. I asked him if he had heard of Dr. Knowals. He said he had and that he thought very highly of him. I said I thought very highly of Dr. Knowals too and, therefore, I would follow his stipulations to the letter.

Dr. Shautt angrily stated that in Tenderloin things are done as he, Dr. Shautt, decrees and not as any other physician stipulates. There had apparently been some misunderstanding, he said, between his assistant and Dr. Legume. Breast surgery in Tenderloin, he said, was done in the main operating room, under general anesthesia, and I would be required to sign a hospital consent form.

Suddenly, he raised his voice and shouted, "Well, hurry up, make up your mind. Are you going to be here on July 1st or not? I'm in a hurry. I'm leaving for my vacation this afternoon."

Since he was not going to conform to Dr. Knowals' stipulations, I certainly was not going to have my surgery performed at Dr. Shautt's hospital. However, I could not resist asking, "If you are going on vacation, who would be performing the surgery?"

"My assistant, Dr. Grafe," he replied.

The name, "Dr. Grafe," brought back some very unpleasant memories. A few years back, Dr. Grafe had operated on someone close to me. After the operation, Dr. Grafe came out of the operating room with a smile on his face and said, "The operation was very successful."

Dr. Grafe was asked when the patient could be seen. Still smiling, he replied, "Oh, you can't see the patient. He went into a coma."

There is the old layman's joke about the operation being successful, but the patient died. When a surgeon speaks this way, it is, to say the least, unconscionable! The patient died a few days later, as Dr. Grafe knew he would! May God have mercy on Dr. Grafe's patients. This surgeon is far more concerned about his pretty stitches (the success of his surgery!) than with his patients' lives!!!

I wanted to bring the conversation with Dr. Shautt to an end. Under no circumstances would I permit Dr. Grafe to operate on me nor would I budge one iota from Dr. Knowals' stipulations, but, when Dr. Shautt, in an irritated state, asked, "Well, will you be here on July 1st or not," I replied pensively, "No, someone close to me died in that operating room."

Dr. Shautt raised his voice in anger to a higher pitch and shouted, "Someone close to you died here! You've gotta die some place. You might as well die at Tenderloin!"

I had to control myself to keep from telling Dr. Shautt what I thought of him. Instead, I quietly said, "Shautt" — (I wouldn't call him "doctor" after what he had just said) — "Shautt, please hurry and go on your vacation, then some people who would otherwise die by your knife will continue to live. It hasn't been pleasant speaking with you. Good-bye, Shautt."

I don't think Shautt heard a word I said. He was too immersed in thoughts of his vacation and couldn't care less about patients.

In the hospital in which Dr. Shautt performs surgery — as in most other "teaching" hospitals throughout the United States — all breast surgery is done in the main operating room with the patient under general anesthesia. While the patient is under this anesthesia, a biopsy of her breast tumor is performed to determine whether or not the tumor is malignant. If the tumor is found to be malignant, a radical mastectomy is performed immediately.

Dr. Shautt recently said to a physician-friend of mine, "Why should women be allowed to enter into any decisions about treatment of their breast cancer?"

Why should women be allowed to enter into any decisions about their breast cancer? *Because it is their breasts, their bodies, and their lives that are at stake!*

I phoned Dr. Knowals that afternoon and told him what had taken place between Dr. Shautt and myself. Dr. Knowals gave me the names of three surgeons whom he considered competent and compassionate and who would follow his stipulations. I chose the one who, for several reasons, I believed would comply with the stipulations with exactitude and in a most competent manner.

The following day, I was examined by this surgeon, Dr. Kandoer. He explained to me exactly where he would make the local incision and how he would perform the surgery. His concern and compassion impressed me. Dr. Kandoer, it was obvious to me, is a surgeon who cares.

On Monday, July 14, 1975, I went to Kitchener Hospital, a private hospital, for the excision of the little lump in my left breast. A little while after I arrived, I was surgically "prep"ed. This consisted of blood tests, chest x-rays, electrocardiogram, and urine analysis. Later, when I was in my room, a hospital nurse approached my bed. She had a hypodermic needle in one hand and a hospital consent form in the other. She gave me the release and a pen and said, "Sign this."

I said, "I'm sorry, but I will not sign a hospital release."

She was stunned. Apparently, no one had ever said this to her before.

Generally, patients are so frightened by the hospital personnel and the entire hospital atmosphere and in such fear of the surgery for which they have entered the hospital that they sign hospital releases without reading a word of what is in the release.

A doctor, nurse or nurse's aide says, "Sign," and, intimidated, the patient signs. The patient, thereby, gives the doctors, nurses and the hospital the right to do whatever they please with the patient — administer any drugs, do any surgical procedure, or perform any test or experiment on the patient.

The nurse stared at me in amazement. "You've got to sign," she said.

"No, I don't."

She left the room. In a few minutes, she returned with the release in her hand. Now, she more firmly stated, "You must sign this."

"No, I must not," I said. "In case you've forgotten," I added, "this is a free country. This is my body. It's the only one I have. And, I shall not sign it away and give you and the hospital and the doctors the right to do as they please with it."

At this point, the nurse picked up the telephone receiver at my bedside, dialed a number, and spoke with the head nurse.

"She refuses to sign," she said into the phone.

Then, she turned to me and said, "The head nurse wants to speak with you."

I took the receiver and heard the voice of the head nurse say, "Dr. Splaver, all you are signing for is what is written in ink."

This consent form, like all releases, was a printed form. Close to the top of the sheet, it states that the surgical procedure to be performed on the patient is . . . . (and there follows a blank space in which the nurse, doctor or other hospital staff member inserts, in ink, the type of surgical or other procedure to be performed). On the form, which I was being asked to sign, "excision of tumor in left breast" was written in ink.

The head nurse repeated, "All you are signing for is what's written in ink."

"Is that so," I said.

"Yes, of course," she said. "The only thing that means anything is what is written in ink," she emphasized. "Don't worry about the printed matter. What's printed doesn't count, only what's written in ink."

I turned to the young woman in white at my bedside and asked her for the release and pen. Thinking I was going to sign, she happily gave them to me. I then proceeded to cross out all the lines of print beneath the inked "excision of tumor in left breast."

The nurse was horrified and shouted, "You can't do that."

"I've done it," I said. "Your head nurse said the printed matter doesn't count, so I crossed it out."

She quickly grabbed the "crossed out" release from my hand and dashed out of the room.

What the head nurse said was an outrageous untruth. Ask any lawyer and you will be told that the only thing that "counts" is the "printed matter". It's what's written in ink that "doesn't count" unless it is initialed by the parties involved. I am confident that the head nurse knew she was lying, or else she had to be very stupid — and I doubt that someone very stupid could rise to the post of head nurse.

About ten minutes later, Dr. Kandoer entered my room and approached my bed. He was followed by the young woman in white who had my "crossed out" release with her.

"You can sign that now," he said with a wry smile on his face.

The nurse gave me this release and I signed it. She left with the "crossed out" release in her hand. I was given an injection and later placed on the stretcher and wheeled out to the operating room. The surgical procedure took about fifteen minutes. I received local anesthesia and, although I experienced no pain throughout the procedure, I was aware of what was taking place.

The surgery performed on my breast was excellent for it was done by an exceptionally competent surgeon. The tumor was small, about one centimeter in size. Although there was hope that it was a papilloma, for safety's sake (in the event that it was malignant), Dr. Kandoer removed the tumor plus some of the healthy tissue surrounding it. Since the tumor was small, even with the excision of some of the surrounding tissue, my breast looks normal. This surgical procedure is popularly called a *lumpectomy* and is technically known as a *tylectomy*.

After I was returned to my room, I was served lunch. I rested in my hospital bed for about three hours after the surgery and then was permitted to go home.

From Monday, July 14th to Friday, July 18th, 1975 was the longest five-day period in my life. On Friday, I was to return to Dr. Kandoer's office at which time he would tell me the results of the biopsy and remove the stitches. It was a beautiful summer day. I walked along Central Park with a song in my heart; even the birds were singing. Buoyed by optimism, I felt very happy and in the best of health.

When I entered the surgeon's examining room, I asked, "What are the results of the biopsy?"

Straightforwardly, he replied, "It's malignant."

I was so stunned, I couldn't believe what he had said. My first reaction was that I was "mirror-hearing" (hearing the opposite or backwards, akin to mirror-writing). I thought to myself, "He said 'benign' and I heard 'malignant'."

Startled, I asked him, "What did you say?"

He repeated, "It's malignant."

This time, it sank in. He had said the dreaded words — and I had heard the dreaded words.

Quickly and compassionately, Dr. Kandoer said, "Don't worry. You'll be all right. There are options available to you. We'll discuss them soon."

Dr. Kandoer removed the surgical tape from my breast and then removed half of the stitches. He said the incision was healing very well. He told me to get dressed and we would then discuss the options. By the time I got dressed and went into his office, the shock had worn off a wee bit.

After I entered his office and seated myself, I berated Dr. Kandoer for telling me the bad news so bluntly. His response was, "But you're a psychologist."

To which I replied, "When you put a knife to my breast, didn't I bleed? Don't you think psychologists feel?"

I added, "Psychologists should feel even more than others or else they shouldn't be psychologists."

Dr. Kandoer thoughtfully said, "I think you have a lot of inner strength. I think the way I told it to you was the best way for you."

When I looked back upon this episode some weeks later, I had no doubt that Dr. Kandoer had done what was best. He is a compassionate man, in addition to being a skilled surgeon, and I have much respect and admiration for him. He was right. I do have a lot of inner strength and it comes primarily from my faith in God.

There has been much controversy as to whether or not a patient should be told that she (or he) has cancer. I believe a patient should be told, but the manner by which she (or he) is told should vary with the individual patient depending upon the patient's general state of health, how much or how little inner strength the patient has, and the prognosis. A patient can do a better job of fighting an illness if the patient knows the truth and if the truth has been told with compassion, caution and hope.

Dr. Kandoer then said, "I will offer you three options. The first option, and this is the one I recommend, is a simple mastectomy."

No sooner was the word "mastectomy" spoken than I said to Dr. Kandoer, "You can discard that option immediately. Under no circumstances would I undergo a mastectomy."

Dr. Kandoer explained that he was not recommending a radical or modified radical mastectomy, but a simple mastectomy. In a simple mastectomy, only the breast is removed. He then explained that according to statistical reports, the chances of my survival might be greater with a simple mastectomy than with the other two options. I told him that I had taken enough statistics courses toward my doctorate to know that with all the variables and unknowns in breast cancer, the statistical reports are quite worthless; additionally, statistics can be so manipulated as to prove whatever one wishes to prove.

As emphatically as possible, I said to Dr. Kandoer, "Under no circumstances would I ever give any physician the right to perform a mastectomy of any kind on me."

I stopped to take a deep breath — it was only a few short minutes since I had heard the words, "it's malignant"— and I continued, "I believe we remain on this earth as long as the good Lord wishes us to remain. As God wants, so shall it be."

Dr. Kandoer stared at me, perhaps in disbelief. Perhaps no other patient had ever said this to him.

"I hope God wants me to stay here for many more years. I want to stay," I added pensively, "but I'll stay with both my breasts."

The stillness in the surgeon's office was almost tangible. I continued, "I am determined to live and I am convinced that my chances of living are better if I do not have a mastectomy. God willing, there will be many years of life ahead of me."

I then asked Dr. Kandoer to please tell me his other two options. The second option he gave me was radiation therapy and the third was wedge resection. The latter involves additional surgery; it consists of more surgery than the tylectomy, but less than the simple mastectomy.

A great deal of credit must be given to Dr. Kandoer. He is a surgeon and is, therefore, surgically oriented. Yet, he recommended a simple mastectomy, not a radical or modified radical mastectomy. This is a significant departure from the "surgical mainstream." He did not even say I "must" have a simple mastectomy. He "recommended" this option over the other two options he offered me.

At this point, Dr. Kandoer's secretary came into his office and gave him a cup of ice cream. He scooped up a spoonful and said, "Here, have some ice cream."

It happened to be my favorite brand. But, I replied, "No, thank you. In all my anxiety this week, I ate too much of that ice cream and gained weight. Now, I have to lose five pounds."

No sooner had I said these words than it all struck me as so ludicrous. I had just been told I had a malignancy and I was concerned about my weight. So, I quickly added, "What the devil am I saying. I may be checking out of Hotel Earth and here I am talking about losing weight. O.K., let's have some of that delicious ice cream."

Dr. Kandoer berated me for what I had just said and admonished, "You're not going to check out for many, many years yet — but, have some ice cream anyway."

"You're right," I said.

My "fighting spirit," which had been partially demolished by the words, "it's malignant," was beginning to return. I had never dodged a challenge and I wouldn't dodge this one either.

"I *am* going to remain on this earth for many more years. I'm going to fight this — and I'm going to win," I told Dr. Kandoer.

My surgeon stuck the spoonful of ice cream into my mouth. I licked off about half of the contents of the spoon. Dr. Kandoer then put the spoon into his mouth and proceeded to eat the rest of the ice cream.

I said, "That's your way of saying cancer is not contagious, isn't it?"

"Of course, it's not contagious," he replied.

Dr. Kandoer said I should return the following Tuesday, July 22nd, for the removal of the remainder of the stitches. In the meantime, he suggested, I should consider the options, discuss them with family and friends, and come to a decision based on my own free will. God bless Dr. Kandoer and surgeons and breast specialists like him — may their tribe increase — who believe that breast cancer patients should have freedom of choice to decide of their own free will which options they prefer.

I told Dr. Kandoer that although I have great respect for him, since this was such a vital decision, I would be doing a lot of discussing with physicians, nurses and others in my family and among my friends, and that I would not come to any decision until Dr. Knowals, my breast specialist, and Dr. Legume, my family doctor, returned. Dr. Legume was away on vacation and would not be back until Wednesday, July 30th. Dr. Knowals was out of the country for professional reasons and would not return to his office until Thursday, July 31st.

As I left Dr. Kandoer's office, he said to me, "You'll be all right. I'm sure you'll make the right decision."

"I'll fight it — and I'll win," I repeated with determination.

Although I was voicing "fighting" words, my knees felt somewhat weak. The words "it's malignant" are the most jarring of words. They shake one up a bit (generally much more than "a bit").

My surgeon looked at me with a worried expression. He asked if I wanted to stay in his office a while longer. I thanked him and repeated his words, "I'll be all right."

The sun was still shining on Fifth Avenue when I emerged from the surgeon's office. But, the day was no longer beautiful and this normally beautiful avenue looked dismal now. The birds that were singing when I entered Dr. Kandoer's office now appeared to be silent. Perhaps they were still singing, but I didn't hear them. Only about an hour had passed, but the world had changed so drastically — my personal world, that is.

The traffic light turned green. I crossed the street. I had several dimes in my change purse. I approached the street telephone booth and called certain close relatives and friends. I also phoned the rabbi of my community's Young Israel Synagogue, told him what had happened, and said I would like to chat with him. Several members of my family and friends had wanted to go with me to the surgeon's office. However, I had been so optimistic that I saw no need for them to take time off from work to accompany me. Now, after hearing the words, "it's malignant," I was sorry I had not permitted at least one person to come along with me. In place of someone, the phone calls I was making were of great help and very valuable to me.

My rabbi is a very erudite, thoughtful man and it was good to chat with him. Actually, I did much more listening than chatting, but I found it very spiritually invigorating and fortifying. I did not stay very long because it was close to the Friday evening Sabbath services and, additionally, I was eager to get home.

When I arrived home, the phones were ringing. The news had spread and the concern of so many friends and relatives buoyed my spirits.

One of the first persons with whom I spoke was a cousin of mine, a young internist, who received his M.D. degree in 1968. After completing his internship and residency in internal medicine, he entered private practice in 1972. My cousin and I are quite fond of each other and he was moved when he heard the news. We discussed all aspects of the situation. He explained the "pro"s and "con"s of radiation therapy and of any further surgery as applied to my specific case.

Thoughtfully, he said, "Sarah, you had a tylectomy. You have an excellent surgeon." (Coincidentally, my cousin attended medical school with Dr. Kandoer's son.)

My cousin continued, "Your tumor was small. It was in an early stage. Chances are excellent that the entire malignancy was removed. You have a fourth option — not to do anything further."

I also discussed my options with my brother-in-law, who is a physician, and he too was helpful.

The next several days, until I would return to Dr. Kandoer's office on Tuesday, July 22nd, for examination and removal of the remaining stitches, were spent discussing, investigating, and reading articles and books on breast cancer. I also talked with other physicians (including surgeons), nurses, and many others who might be in any way knowledgeable about breast cancer.

When I returned to Dr. Kandoer on Tuesday, July 22nd, I told him that my cousin, the internist, had suggested a fourth option. Dr. Kandoer immediately said, "Yes, you have a fourth option. And, that is to do nothing further. But, I wouldn't recommend it."

Breast cancer is a mysterious illness. Sad to say, in this the last quarter of the twentieth century, little is yet known about it and controversy rages. It is, therefore, perfectly proper and possible for honorable, well meaning, knowledgeable medical specialists to have different points of view as to the mode of treatment for individual cases, according to the specialty-orientation of each physician.

Several of my friends had heard of a certain "well-known breast surgeon" in a "well-known medical center" and they were prevailing upon me to visit him for a consultation. I told Dr. Kandoer that this had been suggested to me. He thought this was a good suggestion and told me he would make the biopsy slide, the pathologist's report, the mammograms, and the thermography report available to me.

It is extremely difficult to come to a decision of such importance when even the medical specialists admit that so much about breast cancer is still unknown. Since I would not arrive at any decision until I discussed it with Dr. Legume and Dr. Knowals and they would not be back until July 30th and July 31st respectively, Dr. Kandoer advised me to go for consultation and to gather all the information I could within that period of time.

I phoned Gildnest Medical Center, the "well-known medical center," and spoke with Dr. Pheless, the "well-known breast surgeon." We made an appointment for the following week, Tuesday, July 29th, at 11:00 a.m.

During the week from Tuesday, July 22nd to Tuesday, July 29th, I continued my discussions with medical personnel. I also spent a good deal of time in medical libraries reading many of the medical books and articles on breast diseases.

These books and articles are comprehensible to me for I was a physiology major and biology minor as an undergraduate and have since then kept abreast of medical matters. The sad conclusion is that conflict reigns supreme on the subject of breast cancer. One book contradicts the second book. One article says one thing and the second article says the reverse.

When it is vital to think lucidly, you do not want barriers in your pathway to impede this clear thinking. I am very fortunate that I have many friends and relatives who said and did what was right and thus removed barriers and enhanced my ability to think straight at this difficult time in my life.

There were, too, the well meaning people who said the wrong things; and some well meaning people who were funny, although they did not mean to be so. Yes, strange as it may seem, there can be funny happenings even at a time when a woman learns she was stricken with breast cancer. It is not easy to maintain one's sense of humor after hearing the words, "it's malignant," but it is very important that one does so, for laughter is good "medicine" and helps to reduce the tension.

I have been told that I have a good sense of humor. That is fortunate for me, for I did get a good laugh from the three women, all well intentioned and eager for me to be in good health, who implored me to ask my doctors whether my malignancy was a "he cancer" or a "she cancer". When the first woman asked me, "Is your breast cancer a 'he cancer' or a 'she cancer'?," I was perplexed. I had never heard such nonsense.

I had begun to hear all sorts of strange things about breast cancer (and was destined to hear many more as time went on) — but "he cancer" and "she cancer"!

To the first and second women who asked me this question and who insisted that if I knew whether it was a "he" or a "she" it would be easier to cure, I answered seriously and tried to explain to them that there are no such things as "he cancers" and "she cancers." But, they were insistent and could not understand why I would not ask this question of my doctors.

When a third woman asked me, "Is it a 'he cancer' or a 'she cancer'?" I decided it was pointless to reply seriously. So, I said, "It's not a 'he cancer' or a 'she cancer', it's a 'me cancer'."

She didn't think my reply was funny.

Several other women, also well intentioned, pleaded with me to put jelly on my left breast (from which the tumor had been removed). Here, too, I tried to explain matters scientifically to the first two women who said this to me. By the time the third woman told me to put jelly on my breast, I was very weary and I decided that a touch of humor would be the best approach to this suggestion.

So, I asked, "Raspberry or strawberry?"

She took me seriously and replied, "It doesn't make any difference. Either one."

"But I like grape jelly," I said.

"That's all right too. Put on grape jelly," she replied.

I sometimes wonder where women (and men too) get these strange ideas and misinformation. These are nice people and they mean well. And, they did give me a good chuckle. This was very valuable, for there were not many chuckles for me in the latter half of July 1975.

I could probably fill up a book with odd nostrums which well meaning people told me would "cure" breast cancer. When the medical profession does not know how best to cure a particular illness, the public fills this "vacuum" with "old wives' tales" and quackeries of all types. I will not divulge any of the latter here, for I do not want to take any chances that someone with breast cancer may resort to the use of these worthless nostrums rather than follow the advice of a competent breast specialist.

Mimi Brinkley was quite another matter. She was not well intentioned. When one is stricken with a serious illness and needs to think clearly in order to come to the wisest possible decision, one should put a great distance between oneself and the Mimi Brinkleys of this world.

Mimi Brinkley was an acquaintance, one of many, many acquaintances I have. In June, Mimi had learned that I was going for mammography and other breast examinations and she phoned to ask me about the results. I thought it was nice of her to be concerned. I told her that, on the basis of the test results, the tumor appeared to be benign.

When she said, "Oh," with what sounded like obvious disappointment, I could not believe my ears. But, she caught herself and quickly covered up that "oh" with an, "Oh — I'm glad to hear that."

I could not believe anyone could be so wicked as to be disappointed when an acquaintance's — or, any fellow human being's — tumor "appeared to be benign," so I gave her the benefit of the doubt. Perhaps she was clearing her throat and that was a grunt rather than a disappointed "oh."

I explained to Mimi that since what appears to be a benign papilloma may actually be a cancer, Dr. Knowals had recommended it be removed. I said it would be removed at Tenderloin Hospital on July 1st.

One July 2nd, Mimi phoned thinking I had been operated on the preceding day. I told her what had happened between Dr. Shautt and myself. I was startled when she angrily shouted at me, "Where do you get the nerve to tell a surgeon what to do?"

I told her I was surprised at her reaction.

"What do you mean by 'nerve'!," I said. "It's my body, Mimi. I will not permit a surgeon — or any doctor — to do as he pleases with my body."

Mimi was a well educated woman, the holder of several degrees, who had a position of authority in a public school system. She should have known better. It was obvious that something was troubling Mimi.

She angrily ordered me, "You should go to Tenderloin and have Dr. Shautt give you general anesthesia. Sign the release as everyone does!"

"And as everyone shouldn't!," I retorted.

"Don't you tell me what to do about a tumor in my breast," I continued. "Dr. Knowals is my breast specialist and I'll follow his orders, not yours! Dr. Kandoer will operate on me on July 14th at Kitchener Hospital and he will comply with all of Dr. Knowals' stipulations.

In the evening of Monday, July 14th, Mimi phoned my home to ask about the operation. I was in bed resting after the surgery. When she asked about the biopsy results, she was informed that I would receive them Friday afternoon, July 18th.

She said she was going away for that weekend and would call again on Monday, July 21st.

The following Monday, Mimi did phone again. I answered the phone. Mimi expressed annoyance that she had to call a number of times before she could get through because my phones had been busy. I said I was sorry she had encountered this problem, but I was happy that so many of my friends and relatives were concerned about my health.

Then, she asked, "What were the biopsy results?"

"The news was bad. It was malignant," I replied pensively.

My reply triggered a response that startled me. Mimi expressed no sympathy. Not one word such as, "I'm sorry."

Instead, happily, Mimi shrieked, "Now, aren't you sorry you didn't do the whole job all at once!"

Astonished, I asked, "What job?"

"The mastectomy, of course."

"Who's having a mastectomy?," I asked.

"You!" She shouted this out like the order of a concentration camp guard.

Slowly and calmly, I asked, "Who are you to tell me I am going to have a mastectomy?"

"I know five women who have breast cancer and they all had mastectomies," she replied.

"I know five women who had accidents in which they broke a leg. Must I, therefore, break a leg too?" I asked Mimi.

Her voice began to rise as she replied, "But, you must have a mastectomy."

"For your information, Mimi, I am not having a mastectomy. My malignancy was small and caught in an early stage and, therefore, I do not need a mastectomy."

Mimi obviously had not expected this response from me. She became hysterical and shouted, "You MUST have a mastectomy. You MUST have a mastectomy."

"Don't tell me what I must have," I stated firmly. "You are not a breast specialist. My breast specialist will tell me what to do and then, I'll make the ultimate decision. It's my breast — and my life."

She continued to shout over and over again, even while I was speaking. "You MUST have a mastectomy. You MUST have a mastectomy" . . . and on and on, like a broken record, she continued to shout.

When she stopped to catch her breath, I repeated, "I am not having a mastectomy. You are not my specialist. I have a specialist who will help me decide which option I will choose. And, please, do not bother me any further."

Mimi's hysterical shouts went on. "You MUST have a mastectomy. You MUST have a mastectomy. You MUST have a mastectomy."

I did not hang up on her because I consider it impolite to hang up on someone without saying good-bye. Suddenly, the shouting ceased. She MUST have become exhausted.

I quickly said, "Good-bye, Mimi."

She immediately resumed screaming, "You MUST have a mastectomy."

I raised my voice above her screams. "Good-bye, Mimi," I repeated.

As I replaced the telephone receiver, I wondered how many pills Mimi would be taking to tranquilize herself.

Two nights later, on Wednesday evening, Mimi phoned again. In a very dignified, quiet manner, she said, "Now, don't get excited. Don't get hysterical. I want you to be calm. I have something important to tell you."

She was hysterical two nights earlier and here she was telling me "to be calm."

This is typical of this type of person; she describes her own behavior and attributes it to some other person.

"I went to my doctor today," she continued, "and he told me he knows your breast specialist."

"I'm really not interested in your doctor and anything he has to say," I said.

Her voice rose — and the dignity was gone — as she said, "My doctor called Dr. Knowals and Dr. Knowals told my doctor you MUST have a mastectomy!"

This lie was unconscionable!!!

"Mimi, you should be ashamed of yourself for this outrageous lie."

"It's not a lie. It's the truth. Your breast specialist told my doctor you MUST have a mastectomy," she shouted.

Her lie made me so angry that I now raised my voice as I said to her, "Your doctor didn't speak with Dr. Knowals, because Dr. Knowals is out of the country. And you are a teacher! Do you teach your children to lie too!"

I would like to add here that even if Dr. Knowals had been in the city at that time, UNDER NO CIRCUMSTANCES WOULD HE DIVULGE CONFIDENCES. No ethical doctor would and there are none more ethical than Dr. Knowals!

Being caught in this disgraceful lie, Mimi resorted again to her hysterical shouts, "You MUST have a mastectomy. You MUST have a mastectomy."

"Why are you so anxious for me to have a mastectomy, Mimi?," I asked.

"Because I want you to live." She shouted this lie!

I had had enough of Mimi. I wanted to bring this conversation to an end. Firmly, I said, "YOU want me to live more than my family and friends do! YOU who said 'oh' with such disappointment when I told you there was hope the tumor might be benign! YOU who didn't have the decency enough to say, 'I'm sorry,' when I told you it was malignant, but instead you happily shrieked, 'Aren't you sorry you didn't do the whole job at once.'!"

She wasn't listening to what I was saying. She continued to shriek, "You MUST have a mastectomy."

It was less than a week since I had heard the dreaded words, "it's malignant."

Time was precious. I had so much investigating, so much discussing, so much reading, so much thinking to do, to help me make the wisest possible choice from among the options I had been given. I couldn't allow this emotionally troubled woman to waste any more of my valuable time. The only way to terminate this conversation and prevent any further ones like this was to bring Mimi back to reality. .... ("Know the truth and the truth shall make you free," states the Bible.)

"Mimi, when did you have your mastectomy?," I asked.

This question stunned her back to reality. "Ya — ya — ya — you, you think — I had — a mastectomy," she stammered.

"I don't think so. I know so. You have told me so, by your shouting that I must have a mastectomy."

"Ya — ya — you — think — I want you — to join the club," she continued to stammer.

"Yes," I said. "You had a mastectomy and, therefore, you want me to have a mastectomy." (I have since come to learn that this, unfortunately, is true of the majority of mastectomees. It is, therefore, essential that a woman with a breast disease symptom should *not* consult with a mastectomee, for the mastectomee would, in all probability, do everything to convince her to have a mastectomy too whether the woman needs it or not.)

The silence on the other side of the phone was almost tangible; it was in such sharp contrast to Mimi's previous shrieking and shouting.

"Mimi," I said slowly — and I hope compassionately — "I'm sorry you had a mastectomy. I hope you live in good health for many more years. I will not 'join the club'. You had your options. I have mine. I wish you well. I hope you have the decency to wish me well."

I said good-bye and that ended the conversation. I have since learned — and this is the sad part — that Mimi Brinkley never had any options. She was put under general anesthesia and awoke to the trauma of discovering that her breast had been removed.

The following week, on Tuesday, July 29, 1975, I went to Gildnest Medical Center to consult with Dr. Pheless, the "well-known breast surgeon." My appointment was for 11:00 a.m. The hospital floor nurse asked me to be seated. Thirty minutes passed. I arose and approached the nurses' section. I told the nurse that I was concerned lest I not see the doctor, since it was getting close to twelve noon.

"He leaves at twelve," I said.

The nurse looked puzzled. "Who told you that?"

"Dr. Pheless did," I answered. "When I made the appointment with him last week."

She laughed. "He sees patients all day long. At all hours. He'll see you soon."

In a few minutes, I was ushered into an examining room. A nurse gave me a sheet, told me to get undressed in the adjoining booth, and then left.

At approximately 11:45 a.m., the door opened and in walked Dr. Pheless himself. I have seen many troubled people and many sour and dour facial expressions, but never before had I seen as sour and dour an expression as I saw on this doctor's face. It was as though he had swallowed a container of unsweetened lemon juice all in one gulp.

I said, "Good morning."

He did not reply. I was seated in a chair at the left of Dr. Pheless' desk. As he seated himself, he asked me, "Are you Dr. Splaver?"

"Yes," I replied.

In a very austere manner, Dr. Pheless asked some routine questions. Among other things, he wanted to know the names of my breast specialist and surgeon. I told him. He said he knew them.

I told him that Dr. Knowals was out of the country. Then, I handed him a large envelope. "This contains the mammograms, biopsy slide, and reports that you requested."

He took the envelope and continued to ask questions. "Your mother had breast cancer?," he asked in a manner that indicated he expected a positive reply.

"No, she did not," I replied. "She died a few months ago. She never had breast cancer or any other cancer."

"Who in your family had cancer?"

"No one. I can trace my family back to my great-grandparents," I told him. "No one had cancer, breast cancer or any other form of malignancy."

There are those doctors who believe that there is a genetic basis to cancer, that it "runs in the family." Dr. Pheless seemed disappointed that he could not fit me into this pattern of thought. He asked me to sit on the examining table. He looked at my left breast and palpated it in a very cursory manner. Then, he returned to his desk, picked up the envelope I had given him, and removed one x-ray film. There were five mammograms in the envelope.

Dr. Pheless held the mammogram at arm's length. I watched in astonishment as I noted that his head was turned at about a 30⁰ angle away from the mammogram. He was not at all looking at the film!

He turned to me and the first syllable came forth from his mouth like the bleet of a sheep as he thundered, "Maaaaaaaaa — stectomy!"

"Can you come to that judgment on the basis of looking at just one mammogram?," I asked. (Actually, he hadn't even looked at this one! As I said, his gaze was at least at a 30° angle to the extended arm and hand holding the x-ray film.)

"Don't tell me on what basis to form a judgment," bellowed Dr. Pheless.

As I studied the obnoxious expression on his face, I wasn't quite sure whether to regard this man with pity or contempt.

Suddenly, his words burst forth like the bark of a wild dog as he shouted, "Why do you value your breasts?"

"I happen to be anti-surgery. But," I added, "I could probably write an article in answer to your question. Briefly, I value my breasts for the same reasons that every normal woman values them, for the same reasons every normal man values his genitals."

His facial expression became even more grotesque. Dr. Pheless probably did like my equating male genitals with female breasts. In view of his behavior, I could only conclude that women are even less than second class citizens to him. The coldheartedness, pomposity and arrogance of this physician exceeded anything I had ever encountered.

Unexpectedly, Dr. Pheless roared, "How's your sex life?"

I was on the verge of replying by asking him, "How's yours, doctor?"

However, I wasn't entirely certain whether he was drunk or on some other drug or simply sadistic, so I decided to control my impulse to respond in this manner.

Before I could say anything, he growled, "Do you have a lover?"

This time, I so very much wanted to counter his question with, "Do you have a mistress, doctor?"

I would like to state here that "How's your sex life?" and "Do you have a lover?" are not questions typically asked by breast specialists and surgeons. However, it is not possible to predict what type of questions may come out of the mouth of a Dr. Pheless.

I could not reply to Dr. Pheless for he suddenly left this line of questioning and growled, "Why don't you have a wedge resection?"

I was not sure whether he was making a statement or asking a question. I asked, "Are you recommending a wedge resection?"

He didn't reply to my question, but began to draw pictures illustrating how a wider excision could be made around the area from which my little malignant tumor had been removed. He was drawing a diagram of a wedge resection.

At this point, a younger physician, Dr. Lenfant, entered the room and exchanged greetings with Dr. Pheless. Dr. Lenfant had a smile on his face and this was a welcome contrast to the "ugliness" of Dr. Pheless' face. He asked if he might examine my breasts. I said I had no objection to his doing so. I thought I might get a more professional examination and judgment from Dr. Lenfant than from the troubled Dr. Pheless.

Before Dr. Lenfant could examine me, however, Dr. Pheless pulled him aside and in a whisper loud enough for me to hear said, "She's a patient of Dr. Knowals and Dr. Kandoer. If she had any further surgery, it wouldn't be here."

He then pulled Dr. Lenfant toward the door. As Dr. Lenfant passed the examining table on which I was still perched, he whispered, "I'd like to tell you something."

Dr. Pheless pulled him out of the room and the two disappeared.

I stepped down from the examining table, got dressed, and sat down on the chair alongside of Dr. Pheless' desk. As I sat immersed in thought, I wondered whether the women who spoke highly of Dr. Pheless and Gildnest Medical Center had ever been his patients or had ever been in this hospital. Probably not. Or else, they had been brainwashed, just as women for one hundred years have been brainwashed, to think that every breast malignancy must be followed by a mastectomy.

Ten minutes went by. Fifteen minutes went by. Twenty minutes went by. I wondered where Dr. Pheless had gone and whether he would return. At last, the door opened. It was Dr. Pheless.

"Go to lunch," he ordered, "and be back at 1:30."

I was not in the mood for lunch after this harrowing experience with Dr. Pheless. I had a glass of orange juice, relaxed for a while, and then went back upstairs. When I returned to the examining room, it was 1:30 p.m. It was not until 2:00 p.m. that Dr. Pheless returned.

He seated himself, then turned to me and said, "The pathologist examined your biopsy slide. I have the report."

Suddenly, his face became contorted into a Hitlerian expression as he distinctly spat out each word. "You've — got — the — *real* — thing" — he paused, and with greater emphasis repeated — "the — REAL — thing."

I decided that if this evil man wanted to engage in a verbal wrestling match, I would show him he could not demolish me. Imitating his manner of speech, I said, "If it were not — the — REAL — thing — I would not have come here for a consultation."

"Why don't you go for radiation therapy?," he barked.

I looked at him in a state of puzzlement. I had read an article written by Dr. Pheless in which he was anti-radiation therapy.

"Doctor, in your article you said you were against radiation therapy. Are you now advocating it?," I asked.

"Don't you tell me what I said in my article," he bellowed.

Lowering his voice a bit, he asked me, "What is your opinion? What further treatment do you want?"

"I haven't come to any decision," I replied. "I've spoken to many physicians and ——"

Dr. Pheless startled me with his unexpected interruption. My blood pressure probably rose at least ten points. He had jumped up from his chair and barked at me. "I'm not going to waste my valuable time listening to you tell me what other doctors have said."

Then, he growled, "What is YOUR decision?"

Treating him as though he were emotionally ill — which I believe he was, in addition to being sadistic — I quietly and precisely said, "I am not a breast specialist, nor a physician of any kind. My decision must be based upon what I learn from breast specialists and other physicians. I haven't arrived at any decision as yet. Dr. Knowals is away and won't return until the 31st. That is why I have come here."

This appeared to have calmed him somewhat. He remained standing for a few minutes, and then started toward the door. I followed after him, pleased to be getting out of there.

At the doorway, Dr. Pheless stopped and sternly said to me, "You've had a lumpectomy. What more do you want! You don't have to do anything more — and you could live ten, twenty, thirty or even more years."

Then, he entered the hallway and stalked off without as much as a "good-bye and good luck."

As I started to walk toward the elevator, I remembered that Dr. Lenfant had said he had something to tell me. Before leaving, I wanted to find him and ask him what it was he wanted to tell me. I did not know where Dr. Lenfant was and no one was there to help me find him. So, I proceeded down the hallway, stopping at each open doorway to look into the room in search of Dr. Lenfant. Suddenly, I heard a shriek that surely sent my blood pressure up twenty points this time.

Dr. Pheless was sitting in the room opposite the one at which I had just stopped. When he saw me look inside, he shrieked, "WHAT ARE YOU LOOKING FOR?"

"I'm looking for Dr. Lenfant."

"He's not available."

"He said he had something he wanted to tell me."

Again Dr. Pheless bleeted like a sheep as he sneered, "He wanted to tell you — maaaaaaaaaa — stectomy!"

As I hurried away from Dr. Pheless, it saddened me to think of how many women he had undoubtedly demolished. Many doctors differ with each other as to the best method of treatment of breast cancer. Dr. Pheless differs with himself!

Dr. Legume, my family physician, returned from his vacation the following day, Wednesday, July 30th. That morning, I went to his office and related to him the events that had transpired while he was away. We discussed my situation and he gave me helpful information and advice. I left his office with the understanding that I would return and we would talk some more after I saw Dr. Knowals the following day.

When I entered Dr. Knowals' office the next day, he greeted me with an expression of such compassion that the burden of decision I carried within me immediately became ever so much lighter.

Only two days had passed since I had seen that horrible Dr. Pheless. In Dr. Pheless' face, there was just ugly negative anger, devoid of any compassion. When I think of him, it brings to mind Samuel Johnson's statement, "The wretched have no compassion."

In Dr. Knowals' face, there was such splendid tenderness, supportive strength and serene humanity, which every physician should possess, but few do.

Dr. Knowals explained to me the nature of breast malignancies in general and my malignancy specifically. As he spoke — and I listened — I thanked God that Dr. Legume had referred me to him for I became convinced that the information and advice this kindly, knowledgeable breast specialist would give me would help me to arrive at the right decision. He, with God's help, would help me get well.

Dr. Knowals told me that the prognosis in my case is good. The malignancy was detected early. The tumor was small and was entirely removed in the tylectomy. Despite the additional tissue that was removed for safety's sake, the breast looked normal and the scar had healed well.

Dr. Knowals believes in matching the treatment to the individual case. He said there were three options available to me on the basis of my specific case.

These are the three options offered to me by Dr. Knowals: 1) to do nothing further beyond the tylectomy which had been performed on me and to "watch" the condition via periodic mammography, thermography and clinical examinations; 2) to have radiation therapy, the length and number of treatments to be decided upon after further examination; and, 3) to undergo additional, but limited surgery (wedge resection).

Options no. 2 and no. 3 were the same as the second and third options which Dr. Kandoer, my surgeon, had offered me. Dr. Knowals, the breast specialist, and Dr. Kandoer, the surgeon, differed on option no. 1. Whereas Dr. Kandoer, suggested a simple mastectomy as the first option, Dr. Knowals' first option was to do nothing further. Mastectomy was not included among Dr. Knowals' options; he knew I refused to consider mastectomy as an option.

I want to stress here that this difference of opinion between Dr. Knowals and Dr. Kandoer is perfectly understandable and acceptable. Each of these superb physicians, for whom I have the highest respect, has his own specialty orientation and each, via his orientation, aims to save the lives of his patients. Since so much is unknown about breast cancer and since the medical profession is not in agreement as to what is the best treatment for breast cancer, the treatment suggested by physicians involved with breast diseases may vary according to the perspective of each physician's specialization.

"The ultimate decision must be yours," said Dr. Knowals. "Since so much about breast cancer is still unknown to us, the patient has to be a partner with the physician in deciding on the treatment."

I agree! With an illness such as breast cancer, where so little is known, the patient must have freedom to choose the mode of treatment in her specific case. It is her breast, her body, her life, and not the physician's.

I spent the next day, Friday, August 1, 1975, and the weekend in deep thought, digesting all the information I had gathered from all sources. I took all the time I considered necessary in order to arrive at, what I hoped would be, the best possible decision. A decision of this magnitude is not something at which one can, or should, arrive at in a hurry. It is best not to come to a quick decision.

The subject of cancer is so emotionally charged that all too often people tend to panic and act in haste. They have heard the dreaded word "metastasis" and they live in fear of it. If, God forbid, metastasis has begun, it makes no difference if one hurries with one's decision or if one deliberates. If metastasis has not begun — and, hopefully, never shall — it is much better to take one's time in arriving at a decision, for a decision made in haste is generally a wrong one. With breast cancer, a decision made in haste may lead to excessive surgery or an unnecessary mastectomy.

Dr. Knowals had discussed with me the "pros" and "cons" of each of the options open to me and I gave serious consideration to each of these on, what was for me, that fateful weekend of August 1st-4th, 1975.

Each option had many "pros" and "cons". Each had its dangers. Let us not forget, however, that living is a danger. From the moment we leave our mother's womb, we are in danger of destruction! As a matter of fact, we are in danger even in our mother's womb. There was a story in the papers recently of a pregnant woman who was shot during a robbery. Her life was saved, but the fetus within her was fatally wounded.

So, after all of this deep thought, digesting all I had learned and been told, on Monday, August 4, 1975, I arrived at a decision. I decided to choose option no. 1: to do nothing further beyond the tylectomy which had already been performed on me and to "watch" the condition via mammography, thermography and clinical examinations on a periodic basis.

I arrived at my decision of my own free volition and assume complete responsibility for it. That is the only way it should be for it is my breast, my body, my life. EVERY WOMAN IN A SIMILAR SITUATION MUST HAVE THE FREEDOM TO MAKE THE ULTIMATE DECISION HERSELF.

Many friends and relatives were concerned about what had happened to me and were waiting to hear what I had decided. Since I am an author and writing comes easy to me, I stated my thoughts and explained my decision in a letter. On August 5th, I mailed out approximately 150 xeroxed copies of this letter, which included much that is contained in the preceding pages. I then went away for a much needed rest-vacation.

By the time I returned from my vacation, many people had become aware of my choice of option. A number of people told me they had xeroxed my xeroxed letter and handed out copies to people they knew, who were ill and who, they thought, would benefit from reading my letter. As a consequence, I began to receive many phone calls from people who were suffering from a miscellany of illnesses. Most of the calls were from women who had mastectomies.

The calls from these mastectomees came in at the rate of several per day — and night. A small number praised me and said they admired my "courage". Most, however, were bitter and depressed. They were angry at me for not having had a mastectomy, for not having "joined the club", as they put it. Many hurled curses and obscenities at me; many said they were praying that I should die — *they wanted me to die so they could say I died because I had a lumpectomy. It was useless to try to explain to them that I believe the treatment should match the individual case, that local excision was the treatment that best matched my specific case, and that I love life and want to live and, therefore, chose this as my mode of treatment.*

From that time forward, I truly began to learn what a strange illness breast cancer is and I started to call it the "weird world of breast cancer" — and it has become weirder and weirder with the passage of time.

The mastectomy is a devastating, unacceptable surgical procedure and it saddened me to see what their mastectomies had done to these women. These women had been surgically "prep"ed before their operations. I began to wonder why their surgeons had not seen to it that their patients were also psychologically "prep"ed — psychologically prepared for the surgery and psychologically prepared afterwards to cope with their altered physical states. I became determined to help remedy this situation.

Among the callers, only one gave me her name. That was Anne Ecktigertag. Anne phoned me three times. I know a woman who is a relative of Anne's. The relative said, "The mastectomy means nothing to Anne. She goes places and she's full of life."

This was typically far from the truth. It was quite contrary to what Anne told me.

"Sure, I go places," said Anne. "I went to Europe last year. Every place I go I feel like I'm in hell. I smile in public and I put on an act. Hollywood should give me an Oscar. Hollywood should give all the mastectomees an Oscar. We all smile in public. Buckets of tears are in our bedrooms."

During one call, Anne sobbed quietly for several minutes. In-between the tears came the words, "I'm half woman and half dead. Half woman and half dead. Half woman and half dead."

Over and over again, she repeated this refrain. I stopped her. I told her she was not "half woman," she was "all woman." I also said she was not "half dead": she could be very much alive if she wanted to be and how much alive she would continue to be would depend very much upon her desire to be alive.

I told Anne that I very much wanted to help her. I was convinced that with psychological counseling she could be helped to cope with her problems. I invited her to come to my house. She accepted.

Before she came, her relative said to me, "I saw Anne yesterday. Isn't it wonderful. She told me she was never happier in her life than she is right now."

I understood the meaning of this immediately. The denial of pain is pervasive in our society. Some of the unhappiest people say, "I was never happier in my life."

There are many stressful situations which people cannot accept, so they use their "defense mechanisms" to "protect" themselves. "Denial" is one of the most popular of these mechanisms. Thus, the mastectomee who is unhappy says, "I was never happier in my life." Then, she tranquilizes herself with endless pills. How much better it would be if psychological counseling were made available to her to help her adjust wholesomely to the reality of her situation.

Most mastectomees do not need psychiatric help; they are not mentally ill. They are, in the main, normal women who have undergone a very stressful surgical procedure and, as a consequence, have severe problems with which they find it difficult to cope; psychological counseling would, therefore, be of great help to them. There are, however, some mastectom*ees* (women who had mastectom*ies*) who have become mentally ill due to their mastectom*ies* (the surgical procedures); they have fled from reality and do need psychiatric help.

Anne visited me a few days later. However, I soon realized she had not come to be helped. She came to try to convince me that I should have a mastectomy.

"Go for a mastectomy. Join us," she begged me. "Then, you'll be one of us. You can speak; you could help us."

I told her I would be glad to help — but NOT by having a mastectomy, which I do not need. She had read my letter of August 5th and she knew of my choice of option and decision. I said that since my malignant tumor was detected early, a mastectomy was not necessary in my case. I told Anne I was planning to form a health association concerned with breast diseases, just as there are heart, lung and other health associations. It would be called the Breast Diseases Association of America (BDAA).

The BDAA, I explained to her, would strive to educate the women of America about the nature of breast diseases and the importance of early detection. It would fight to eradicate breast cancer. I informed Anne that BDAA hopefully would have a psychological division to offer counseling to mastectomees and others who might need this help. I asked her if she would join in helping to form the Breast Diseases Association of America.

"Of course not," she replied and began to cry.

Anne did not want breast cancer to be eradicated. She wanted more women to be stricken, more women mastectomized, more women to "join the club." Sad to say, there are ever so many mastectomees who feel as Anne does. They believe the worst (mastectomy) has already happened to them. Deep down within them, they live in fear of metastasis and many have daughters who are now more vulnerable to breast cancer. Yet, they have become so emotionally devastated by their radical surgery, they do not want breast cancer to be conquered; their main desire is for more women to "join the club."

Anne left my house when she realized that I would not "join the club."

There were numerous mastectomees who phoned me at 5:00 a.m. and 6:00 a.m. and what they said generally went like this: "I know you can't sleep. I can't sleep either. I want to talk with you."

These callers did not at all "know" that I "can't sleep." They did not know me at all. If they had known me, they would have known that I was sound asleep. I am a very sound sleeper and rarely ever have trouble falling asleep. This is due to the fact that I believe one should not flee in fright from one's problems, but should face them and fight to conquer and cope with them favorably.

I never told these mastectomees that they had awakened me for I sympathized (and could, to a great degree, emphathize) with them. Talking is therapy and I felt that if talking with me would help them I had no objection to their talking even at those early hours, at a time when I needed the sleep and rest. Uniformly, they bemoaned their disfigurement and altered physical states. Then, invariably, they switched their lines of talking and cursed me for not having had a mastectomy.

Toward the end of September 1975, a few days after the mugging incident which I related at the start of this Part, I flew to the home of my wonderful friends, Eve and Al Chaiken, who live near the prestigious Samson Cancer Center. I had appointments to see some of the doctors at Samson.

As the author of many books, I was planning to write a book on my experiences and on lesser surgery as treatment of early breast cancer. I wanted to chat with oncologists at Samson to discuss my case and their attitudes toward lesser surgery in breast cancer treatment.

The controversy which rages on the subject of treatment of breast cancer was probably nowhere as well demonstrated as by what happened to me at the prestigious Samson Cancer Center. Dr. Gilgull and Dr. Emmis are both oncologists specializing in breast cancer. Both had been informed that I had a tylectomy.

I saw Dr. Gigull first. He is a young man, probably in his mid-thirties. As I entered his office, he did not rise, but condescendingly asked, "What do you want?"

"Do you mind if I sit down?," I asked.

He nodded. I sat down. He repeated, "What do you want?"

I said, "I've come for the purpose of getting your views on lumpectomy — tylectomy — "

I stopped abruptly. A strange, guttural sound came out of Dr. Gilgull.

Perhaps the words "lumpectomy" and "tylectomy" had upset him. I thought he was going to throw up.

When he was quiet again, I continued. "I came to get your views on lumpectomy — or, tylectomy, or local excision, as you may call it — and to find out what is new here relative to a possible breakthrough in the treatment of breast cancer."

"Have you got breast cancer?," he asked.

He had been informed that I had a tylectomy. I now re-informed him. "In July, I had a tylectomy in which a small malignant tumor was removed from my left breast."

Dr. Gilgull then proceeded, in a pompous fashion, to make a speech which sounded as though he were reading from a textbook. On and on he went with his overbearing speechifying. I listened politely until I heard him say, "More than fifty per cent of the women with breast cancer are dead within five months of diagnosis of their cancer in spite of their mastectomies. One hundred per cent are dead within five months if they didn't have a radical mastectomy."

"Where do those statistics come from, Dr. Gilgull?," I asked.

Anger suffused his face as he ordered, "Don't interrupt me when I'm speaking."

I listened silently as he continued his contrived dissertation on the benefits of the radical mastectomy. And then, he stopped to catch his breath. This gave me the opportunity to repeat my question.

"Dr. Gilgull, where did you get your statistics?"

"I don't have to answer that question," he snapped.

He didn't have to — that's true — but more important, he couldn't answer. What he had said were lies!

This arrogant, self-proclaimed god then asked, "What's the matter? Can't you face up to your own death? If you don't want to face the truth, that you'll be dead by December 14, 1975, that's your problem.

"We face the truth here," he continued. "You'll die in the fourth or fifth month after your cancer was diagnosed. If you want to deny the truth to yourself, that's up to you."

I laughed in his face to indicate to him how much his prediction meant to me. This angered him.

"Are you giving me only two and a half more months to live, Dr. Gilgull?," I asked.

"Yes," he snapped.

Dr. Gilgull's prediction of my (according to him) impending death did not bother me one iota. I have a deep belief in God and believe it is only God who decides when we leave this earth, not Dr. Gilgull or the likes of him!

What did anger me is that Dr. Gilgull probably has caused many women to undergo mastectomies by frightening them into believing that they will soon die if they do not have these mastectomies. Let a traditionalist surgeon tell a woman she will die tomorrow unless he does a supra-radical mastectomy (mutilation of mutilations!) on her and, totally frightened, she will consent to it.

I looked Dr. Gilgull straight in his eyes and said, "Doctor, I can face the truth. The truth is that you do not possess any God-given powers to predict when I or anyone else will die. I am not afraid to die. But, I plan to live for many, many more years.

I stopped for a moment. Again, he made that strange guttural sound. I thought he might want to say something, but he didn't.

So, I continued. "The truth, Dr. Gilgull, is that we are all going to die ultimately. What about you, doctor? You asked me if I can face the truth. Can you face the truth? Dr. Gilgull, some day you too are going to die."

The latter sentence inflamed him. His lips twitched and his face glowed with anger as he said, "All you're concerned about is your feminine sexuality. Your breasts are so precious to you!"

When a man makes this sort of derogatory remark about a woman's sexuality, it means he is very troubled about his own masculine sexuality.

"Of course my breasts — and my life — are precious to me. And I'll protect my breasts and my life," I emphasized.

"But," I continued, "perhaps it's your masculine sexuality that's bothering you, Dr. Gilgull. Perhaps that's why you are so eager to amputate women's breasts."

"I don't have to listen to this," he "harrumphed" as he rose from his chair and stamped out of the room.

I followed him out of the room and called to him.

He turned around. "Yes?"

"Dr. Gilgull, how about one orchiectomy for each mastectomy?"

The color of his cheeks could have stampeded a herd of bulls. He ran down the hall and out of sight. Apparently, what's good for the goose is not good for the gander. ("Orchiectomy" is the technical term for the excision of the testicles.)

Dr. Emmis' office is a little way down the hall from Dr. Gilgull's office. When I entered Dr. Emmis' office, he rose and asked me to be seated. He asked how I have been feeling since my tylectomy.

"I have been feeling very well, thank God," I informed him.

Dr. Emmis, who is about the same age as Dr. Gilgull, shook his head in approval. "That was very smart of you, having a tylectomy."

"I can't take the credit for it," I said. "The one who is very smart and who deserves the credit is my breast specialist, an exceptionally knowledgeable and compassionate physician."

"You're lucky to have him," said Dr. Emmis. "You'll be all right and you'll live to be 100 because of him, because you had a tylectomy instead of a mastectomy."

Dr. Emmis favors lesser surgery. He told me about the radiation therapy and chemotherapy studies being conducted at Samson Cancer Center.

"The day will come," he said, "when these therapies will replace surgery in the treatment of breast cancer."

"Let's hope that day is not far off," he added.

I asked Dr. Emmis, "How much basis is there for optimism?"

"I think there's good basis," he replied, "but, it's impossible to say when."

We both hoped it would be in the very near future so that no woman would ever again lose her breasts or her life to breast cancer.

As we shook hands in parting — he had to see a patient and I had an appointment with another doctor — Dr. Emmis repeated what he had said earlier.

"You'll be all right. You'll live to be 100 and you'll be all right."

Here were two oncologists at a prestigious cancer center. One told me I would be dead by December 14, 1975 at the latest. The other said I would be all right and live to be 100.

Who's right? Obviously, not Dr. Gilgull! I will not be dead by December 14, 1975, because December 14, 1975 is long gone and I am alive, very much alive, and, thank God, feeling very well. I doubt if I will live to be 100 as Dr. Emmis said I would; but, who knows, perhaps I may! I had great-grandparents who lived past 100.

I believe Dr. Emmis is the knowledgeable oncologist. He has no vested interest in radical breast surgery and he is, as the expression goes, telling it like it is.

On October 3, 1975, shortly after I returned from my visit to Samson Cancer Center, the phone rang loud and clear early in the morning. I picked up the receiver and said, "Hello."

A female voice, unrecognizable to me, asked, "Is this Dr. Splaver?"

I replied, "Yes," and asked the caller who she was.

She ignored my question and said, "I had a mastectomy. Somebody told me you had a lumpectomy."

"I hope you are feeling well," I said and then again asked her, "What is your name, please?"

Again, she ignored my question and went right on talking. "Somebody told me you are anti-mastectomy."

"Then somebody told you wrong," I said. "I am for early detection and for treatment that matches each individual case."

I was not going to allow myself to be drawn into any further discussion on this, or any other, subject, without knowing with whom I was speaking and so I added, "You know who I am. Would you please tell me who you are?"

In reply, she shouted, "I hope you die," and slammed down her receiver.

I stood there for a moment with my receiver in hand and felt so sad for this woman. What would it profit her if I were to die? Nothing! *Were I to die tomorrow, it would still not disprove the fact that tylectomy is an effective mode of treatment for early breast cancer.*

To this woman and to all others who feel as she does, I would like to tell this little tale.

At the time when Dr. Jonas Salk produced the vaccine against polio, I was doing rehabilitation counseling with some disabled young people. The day the newspapers announced the Salk vaccine, the father of a boy disabled due to polio said to me, "That bastard Salk, he should go to hell."

I said to this father, "What would it profit your son if more and more young people were annually disabled by polio?"

He did not reply and so I continued, "What would it profit you if more and more parents would suffer because their children became disabled by polio?"

Again, he did not answer. He had no answers to either question. He was just so full of hostility and frustration, which bring on a state of misery and misery, unfortunately, loves company.

I said to this father, "Let us do all we can to rehabilitate your son. And, let us bless, not curse, Dr. Salk for what he has done."

So, similarly, I ask the woman who called me on October 3, 1975 and all the others who have hurled curses at me because I did not have a mastectomy, "What would it profit you if I were to die?"

Nothing! Nothing at all!

On that day, October 3rd, I decided I did not want to waste any further precious time listening to vicious and/or deranged callers hurling curses, insults and obscenities at me because I chose not to have a mastectomy. Therefore, the following day, I attached phone answering devices to my telephones. Interestingly, these devices did not discourage these callers. They continued and hurled their verbal garbage into the cassettes of the phone answering devices. It is now three years since I installed these devices and some of the weirdest messages have come out of these cassettes.

On Thursday, October 9, 1975, I returned to Dr. Knowals' offices for my first tri-monthly check-up. I had mammography and thermography examinations. Dr. Knowals performed the clinical examinations and reviewed the mammograms and the thermography results.

"Everything is all right," he said.

Happiness is when your breast specialist says, "Everything is all right."

I was told to return in January 1976 for my next tri-monthly examinations.

One morning in November, as I entered a local supermarket to do some shopping, I noticed a woman standing near the doorway, flaying her arms to and fro. She weighed at least 250 pounds, which is twice my weight, and was at least a head taller than my five feet one. As a shopper passed by her, this woman hit the shopper in the face. The shopper quickly ran out of the store.

I had come to buy some paper products. Fortunately, these items were on the shelves of the fifth aisle of the supermarket and, therefore, as far away as I could possibly get from this disturbed woman. Since it was early in the morning, there were few shoppers in the store.

I went to the fifth aisle and proceeded to remove from one of the shelves the boxes of the name brand facial tissues which I generally purchase. As I turned to place these boxes into the cart — POW! — this amazon was facing me and smashed her fist into my right breast. Almost immediately, the manager and two other men pounced on the woman and took her away.

She had not hit me in the left breast on which the lesser surgery had been performed. But, I was very concerned about any trouble she might have caused my right breast. When I returned home, I examined this breast and found a circular black-and-blue area about the size of a quarter on my breast. I phoned my breast specialist and told him what had happened. He told me to come to his office. After he examined my right breast, he informed me that it was a typical black-and-blue bruise from a blow to the breast and that it would gradually diminish and disappear. We "watched" it and in a few weeks, as he had said, the breast was back to normal.

Many people have the false impression that cancer may result from a blow to the breast. This is not so. Although the cause(s) of breast cancer is not known, it is known that a blow on the breast is not a cause. If a woman is accidentally hit in the chest, she normally would examine her breasts to see if any "damage" was done. As a consequence of this examination, she may discover a lump and may think it was caused by the blow. Cancer specialists believe this lump was there long before this woman received the blow, but she had not been examining her breasts before this and, therefore, was unaware that she had a lump in her breast. However, a blow on the breast is a frightening experience for all women.

I have already told you the tale of Gildnest Medical Center, that "well-known medical center" and its "well-known breast surgeon," Dr. Pheless. Let me tell you about my experiences, in December 1975, with Grossum Medical and Cancer Center. It really is "gruesome," but because of the publicity it has received women with breast cancer naively flock there — generally, much to their later regret.

Dr. Rex Zulick is a "well-known breast surgeon" at this "well-known medical center." I have yet to meet anyone as woman-hating as Dr. Zulick. A staunch advocate of the radical mastectomy, he believes that the radical mastectomy should be performed on every woman with even the slightest tumor in one of her breasts, with even the earliest of breast cancer.

When I asked him how he justified radical surgery, a "treatment" which, he admits, has resulted in no reduction in the breast cancer mortality rates in more than forty years, he replied, "We save women's lives by doing radical mastectomies."

In view of the rising mortality rates, his statement is questionable. There are many physicians who say that if the radical mastectomy were abandoned, the mortality rates from breast cancer would fall.

Dr. Zulick told me he would have his nurse phone me the following day to give me the "woman's point of view" toward the radical mastectomy.

I told him, "I'm a woman. It isn't necessary for your nurse to give me the woman's point of view. The woman's point of view toward the radical mastectomy," I added with emphasis, "is that it is a very unacceptable surgical procedure."

He insisted that he wanted his nurse to phone me. The following day, I received a phone call frm Hetta Mayreh, R.N., Dr. Zulick's nurse. She went into a lengthy speech about the benefits of the radical mastectomy, parroting everything that Dr. Zulick had said. I politely interrupted her and told her that I had neither the time nor the desire to listen to a repeat of what Dr. Zulick had said the previous day.

Nurse Hetta Mayreh then said, "If I had breast cancer, I'd have a radical mastectomy because I want to live."

"That's exactly why I had a tylectomy," I retorted, "because I want to live."

Angrily she responded, "Dr. Zulick told me to call you, but I don't know why. What is it you want?"

"You phoned me. I didn't phone you," I said. "I don't know what it is that *you* want."

"Well, what do you want?," she again asked angrily.

Since July, after I heard the words "it's malignant," I had been spending a great many hours in reading the articles on breast diseases in the latest medical and scientific journals, interviewing physicians and surgeons, visiting hospitals and cancer centers, and in other ways investigating what has been happening to breast cancer patients throughout the United States and the world.

I started to say to Nurse Mayreh, "I am gathering information about doctors' attitudes ————— " but she didn't let me finish the sentence.

Her reaction to my words "gathering information" was like that of a bull to a red scarf. I still can't understand why the words "gathering information" disturbed her so much.

With mounting hostility, she said, "You're not going to quote me. I won't let you."

Then, she shouted, "Why didn't you tell me you were gathering information!"

"Quote you!," I said in astonishment. "Why should I quote you? You haven't said anything of value. All you've done is parrot Dr. Zulick's and Grossum's standard policies."

She paid no attention to what I said and began shouting hysterically, "I'm not afraid of you. I shouldn't even be talking to you. I'm busy."

She stopped for a moment to catch her breath and shouted again. "Don't use my name. I won't let you. You don't scare me."

I told her I saw no purpose in continuing this bizarre conversation.

She shouted again, "Don't use my name. Don't quote me, I'm not afraid of you" and then slammed down her telephone receiver.

I believe Hetta Mayreh's hysterics were caused by the fact that she has a fear of being uncovered for what she is. I have reason to believe that Hetta Mayreh is ripping off Grossum and working far less hours than the hours for which she is being paid. She is taking no chances of losing her soft job and, therefore, repeats like a parrot whatever Dr. Zulick says and whatever is the policy of Grossum.

In January 1976, I returned to Dr. Knowals' offices for my second tri-monthly examinations. Thank God, I was told that all was well and that now I need not return again until six months later.

Throughout 1976, I continued my breast cancer investigations. I began to find that there are other surgeons, like my surgeon, who are emotionally stable, who respect women, and who harbor no hostility toward them.

Dr. Fulderman is the director of surgery at a large hospital. When I told him that a tylectomy had been performed on my left breast and gave him information about the tumor, he said, "Good for you. There is excellent likelihood that you will live out your normal life span."

He continued, "We do tylectomies here. We also do wedge resections, simple mastectomies, modified radicals, and radical mastectomies. None of the surgeons here are happy about — as you put it — 'mutilating' — women."

He was referring to the fact that I, earlier in our conversation, had stated that I consider the radical mastectomy an "unacceptable, mutilating surgical procedure."

He spoke with deep feeling as he said, "I have no desire to mutilate any woman. But, at times, we have no choice but to do a radical in an attempt to save the woman's life."

Dr. Fulderman continued to explain that by the time many women go to their physicians, their tumors are large and the malignancy has spread into the auxillary lymph nodes. "In these cases, we have no choice other than radical surgery," he said.

"We do biopsies in our out-patient department," he explained. "If the tumor is malignant, we discuss it with the patient, tell her what we recommend, and let her go home and discuss it with her family. In this way, we reduce some of the trauma of the loss of her breast. It's difficult to fight an illness when the patient is in a traumatized state."

I told Dr. Fulderman about the Breast Diseases Association of America which was in the process of formation. I explained to him what we hoped to accomplish by means of BDAA.

"If you will educate the women of America to practice monthly breast self-examination and to have annual mammography, thermography and clinical examinations," said Dr. Fulderman, "you will be helping to save the lives and the breasts of thousands of women. With early detection, we will be able to do lesser surgery. Just as in your case, where tylectomy was sufficient.''

Not long after my tylectomy, I told Dr. Knowals that I planned to form a health association to disseminate information about breast diseases to the women of America, to foster research to find the cause(s), cure and prevention of breast cancer, and to provide psychological counseling to women stricken with breast diseases, benign as well as malignant. He said he would help in every way possible and he has kept his word.

Several friends of mine and I became the Organizing Committee of the Breast Diseases Association of America (BDAA). During October and November of 1975, members of the Organizing Committee met to discuss and plan the formation of BDAA. In December, we decided we would like to hold a general meeting and I started to look for a meeting room in a suitable New York City midtown location.

I was truly surprised at all the barriers I encountered in the search for a meeting room. I spent hours and days and weeks and months — yes, it ran into months — speaking on the phone and in person to so many people who had the authority to make a meeting room available to BDAA. Time after time, I was given such ''phony'' excuses — often such stupid excuses that one could readily see right through them. Not only did people *not want to aid* in the fight against breast cancer, they wanted *to prevent the fight against breast cancer!* Incredible — yes, incredible — but, also true!

The greatest surprise of all was the commercial ''women's'' organization with available meeting rooms that gave me the biggest and shabbiest ''run-around.'' Some of the women on the staff of this organization became so confused (because they did not want to be involved in the fight against breast cancer and, of course, they did not want their women customers to know this!) that they stalled and stalled, then gave one lame excuse for denying us one of their rooms, and then phoned ten days later with an entirely different lame excuse. Both excuses were such transparent lies, it was absolutely disgraceful!

I believe the women of America should give a great big ''Thank you'' to the Director of Health Education of the Y.M.C.A. who, in March 1976, cordially agreed to make a large room plus many other facilities of the ''Y'' available to BDAA for its first general meeting. We also received fine cooperation from some radio programs and newspapers. Invitational letters were immediately sent out to many women and men who we believed would be interested in fighting breast cancer.

The first general meeting of the Breast Diseases Association of America was held on Saturday, April 24, 1976, at the Y.W.C.A., Lexington Ave. and 53rd St. in New York City. The meeting was attended to capacity by men as well as women and was a resounding success.

From April 24, 1976 forward, the ''weird world of breast cancer'' that I had entered in July 1975 became weirder and weirder. There were so many phone calls from strange people (all women, incidentally) shouting obscenities, insults, curses, and threats into the cassettes of my phone answering devices. These devices have a ''listen-in'' button and I do not speak with callers until they identify themselves; thus, I do not have to waste precious time with strange callers. They, therefore, spewed their venom into the cassettes.

"Drop dead together with the Breast Diseases Association" was an expression to which I became very accustomed, since so many disturbed callers shouted it into the cassettes.

Unquestionably, the strangest of calls was one I received from a noted mastectomee. When she identified herself, I removed the telephone receiver from its cradle and began speaking with her. Her voice exuded hostility from the very start of our conversation, but she was under control for her first few sentences.

Suddenly, she started to shout, "Go fight diabetes. Fight heart disease. Fight headaches. Leave breast cancer alone. Women need breast cancer."

Her last sentence almost stunned me into silence. In consternation, I repeated, slowly and precisely, in questioning manner, "Women need breast cancer?"

"Yes," she shouted, "women need breast cancer. Leave breast cancer alone. Stop the Breast Diseases Association, you God damn bastard!"

She stopped to catch her breath and then shouted, "Go to hell, you God damn bastard" and bang went her telephone receiver.

I have heard many weird remarks since I have been immersed in the "weird world of breast cancer" but her "women need breast cancer" has been truly the weirdest.

In July 1976, six months after my January check-up, I returned to Dr. Knowals' offices for my breast examinations. Thank God, Dr. Knowals said, "Everything is all right."

On Friday, August 20, 1976, after many months of a great deal of "groundwork" activities, the first meeting of the Board of Directors of the Breast Diseases Association of America was held in the office of the Medical Adviser of BDAA. This fledging health association declared its aims to be essentially education, research, and patient care. The legalization process began and in November 1976, BDAA became a legally approved voluntary health association.

Breast cancer is a strange illness. There is no other illness — only breast cancer — where there are so many varied vested interests that do not want that illness to be conquered. I can cope very well with stress. I was able to cope with the plethora of character assassination, curses, insults and obscenities that came through my phones at all hours of the night and day from the summer of 1975 through the summer of 1976 — all caused by the fact that: 1) I did not have a mastectomy, and, 2) I came out fighting against breast cancer. My mammograms were negative in July 1976.

After the first Board of Directors meeting of the Breast Diseases Association of America on August 20, 1976, the harassment and humiliation to which I was subjected by persons who want breast cancer to continue unabated were difficult to contend with for they were so intense and came from such unanticipated sources. From the mouths of "lovely ladies" who want to perpetuate breast cancer came verbal filth the likes of which even truck drivers might be ashamed to use.

When I went for my semi-annual check-up on January 6, 1977, I was quite worried, for I knew what I had endured in the preceding six months, and, therefore, knew that my mammograms might be positive. And, so it came to be on Thursday, January 6, 1977, Dr. Knowals told me that changes had taken place since July 1976. It was a recurrence detected very early and I was to have another tylectomy.

On Friday, January 7th, Dr. Kandoer, my surgeon, examined me and arranged for me to undergo surgery on Wednesday, January 12th at Orello Hospital. Prior to January 6th, so many people had been telling me how "wonderful" and "healthy" I looked. I couldn't have felt more "wonderful" and "healthy." What may puzzle many people is how a woman can look wonderful and feel wonderful and yet have a malignancy within her. The answer is that the malignancy was detected in its very early state.

My brother, Julie, brought me to Orello Hospital's Admitting Office at 10:00 a.m. on Wednesday, January 12, 1977; the surgical "prep"ing had been done the previous day. A woman from Admitting escorted me to my room. It was a room for four. There were two patients in it; one, an elderly woman, Olive, told me she had a "heart condition" and the other, a middle-aged woman, Isabel, said she had diabetes.

Isabel introduced herself, looked at me perplexed, and asked, "What are you doin' here? You look healthy. You walk healthy. You're smilin'. You're healthy. What are you doin' here?"

She looked like she needed cheering up, so I enlarged my smile. Someone once told me, if you must do something you might as well do it with a smile; so, this "anti-surgery" patient was determined to have surgery (lesser surgery, that is) with a smile. Then, I said to Isabel, "Well, a person can look healthy and have cancer."

Isabel obviously superstitious, quickly said, "Don't say that. Don't say that."

"Well, it may be true in my case. And I have to face reality. So, I am saying it," I said.

Isabel wanted to know what was the matter. I told her I was going to have some "problem" removed from my breast. Sadly, she said, "Oh, you're going to have a mastectomy."

The brainwashing of women, for the past 100 years, with the myth that a breast "problem" must be followed by a mastectomy has been so intense and pervasive that Isabel's reaction was typical.

"No," I said. "I'm not going to have a mastectomy. Just the 'problem' removed." Then, I added, "It was detected early. I do not need a mastectomy and I would not permit a mastectomy." (That was all that I said about mastectomy. Read on and you will get a good laugh, I hope, out of how Isabel distorted these statements.)

Isabel jumped up from her chair happily. I thought she was going to do a jig. She shouted, "Boy, you're beautiful. Good for you." Then she turned to Olive and said, 'Ain't she beautiful. She's not gonna have a mastectomy."

At this point, a nurse entered. I was standing by the bed near the door, which I preferred to the other available bed. The nurse gave me a hospital gown and told me to get undressed. Just then a woman (wearing some sort of hospital gown) entered and approached the bed. This woman looked ill. I quickly concluded that this must be her bed and the other bed, which was available, was for me.

So, I said to her, "I'm terribly sorry. I didn't mean to take your bed. I'll go over there."

Angrily, this woman said, "You're the patient, not me. I'm a nurse's aide."

I was so embarrassed at my error, I started to apologize, but she stomped out. As I proceeded to get into the hospital gown and get into bed, Isabel and Olive laughed hysterically.

Isabel said, "You're right. She looks sick. You look healthy."

Olive started to bless me and say some prayers in Latin. I thought this was very nice of her, so, to cheer her up, I told her and Isabel some hospital jokes. They both laughed and laughed. Isabel said, "You're beautiful. Boy, are we glad you're here. You're just what we needed."

I thought, she may be "glad", but I'm not!

A minute or so later, Dr. Knowals entered the room. He said he didn't need to know what room I was in; he heard my laughter down the hallway and followed the laughter.

Then came the surgery. With local anesthesia, I was able to converse with Dr. Kandoer throughout the surgical procedure. Toward the end of the surgery, he said, "Sarah, you're a good patient."

In truth, it's not that I was a "good patient," it is that Dr. Kandoer is an excellent surgeon and I have complete faith in him. When this anti-surgery patient calls a doctor "an excellent surgeon," he must be a "super-excellent surgeon."

The surgery was over and I was returned to my room. I felt very weak and all I wanted to do was to sleep. But, it was visiting hours and Isabel had a visitor. The nurse had pulled the curtain around my bed, but I could hear Isabel saying to her visitor, "Do you know what she said?"

I was determined to hear what I had "said" and so I made an effort not to fall asleep.

Isabel continued, "Boy, she's beautiful. God bless her. She said ______" and suddenly I heard a BANG — (I think she slapped her hand on the bed). I continued to listen intently to hear what I had "said." Then it came.

Isabel's voice rose as she said, "She said, 'I'll die with my busts on'."

Again, there was a BANG. Isabel's voice rose again, " 'I'll die with my busts on'."

There was a third BANG as Isabel shouted out, " 'I'LL DIE WITH MY BUSTS ON' SHE SAID. ISN'T THAT BEAUTIFUL!"

I don't know whether or not that's "beautiful" — I do know I never said it! But weak as I was, I began to laugh. I have been misquoted for many reasons so many times on the subject of mastectomy, since the summer of 1975, but this was the first time that a "misquote" gave me a good laugh.

I was too weak to listen further and fell into a deep sleep. About an hour later, a nurse awakened me and pulled back the curtain. She asked if I wanted anything. I asked her for some orange juice. I must say the service at Orello Hospital was absolutely excellent and everyone with whom I came into contact couldn't possibly have been any nicer.

Isabel and Olive asked me how I felt. I said I felt well, except very weak. Isabel's visitor was still with her. Now, Isabel said to her visitor, "Boy, you think she's beautiful. You should see her doctor. Is he beautiful!"

When Dr. Knowals visited me before the surgery, I jestingly said, "Dr. Knowals, do you think I'll drop dead on the operating table?" And, Dr. Knowals replied, with a straight face, "How can you 'drop dead,' you'll be lying down."

Now, Isabel was telling her visitor, "Boy, what a beautiful doctor. He told her, 'You can't drop dead, you'll be layin' down'."

Over and over again, she kept repeating this statement and roared hysterically as she said it. I was really too weak to laugh and the dressing and bandages made it difficult to laugh, but laugh I did.

Since Isabel thought Dr. Knowals and I were so funny, I said to her, "As soon as I get out of here and get stronger, my doctor and I are forming a comedy team, the comedy team of Splaver and Knowals."

I could have said "Smith and Dale," for she did not know our last names, but she roared with laughter.

Not long thereafter, my brother, Julie, came to get me. At 4:30 p.m., I was discharged and we left for home.

Two days later, on Friday, January 14th, I again heard the dreaded words, but this time Dr. Knowals was there and so too was my brother, Julie, in addition to Dr. Kandoer, and they all helped to ease the blow.

A metastic work-up followed. This involves scanning of various areas and organs of the body to determine whether or not metastasis has occurred. The results, thank God, were negative.

I said in the summer of 1975 — and I say again — that were I to die tomorrow it would not disprove the fact that lumpectomy is an effective mode of treatment for early breast cancer. It saddens me to report that during the one-year period from the time I was first stricken with breast cancer (namely, from July 1975 through June 1976), I knew eleven women who were stricken with breast cancer. All eleven had radical surgery. All eleven are now dead. It saddens me too to report that Mimi Brinkley, whom I mentioned earlier in this Part, is also dead; she died sixteen months after her radical surgery. My recurrence occurred eighteen months after I was first stricken in July 1975.

I shall not "die with my busts on" as my hospital roommate, Isabel, misquoted me. I am determined that I SHALL LIVE WITH MY BREASTS FOR MANY, MANY MORE YEARS. Many physicians have told me that had I had radical surgery in July 1975, as most traditionalist surgeons would have wanted, I would now be long dead.

In July 1975, I had *only* local excision. My recurrence in January 1977 was treated by local excision followed by radiation therapy and chemotherapy. Both times, this is the way I wanted it. Both times, this is the treatment that best matched my individual case.

I believe it is true that "God works in mysterious ways His wonders to perform." Perhaps, it was destined that I should have my recurrence and, therefore, have radiation therapy and chemotherapy. These forms of treatment are extremely unique and, having experienced them, I have a personal, first-hand perspective of the three orthodox modes of cancer treatment, namely, surgery, radiation therapy and chemotherapy. I am, therefore, now much more qualified to be of help to other cancer patients, most of whom have had radiation therapy and/or chemotherapy in addition to surgery.

On the basis of all that I have read and all that I have learned from discussions with many knowledgeable physicians, I am positively inclined toward radiation therapy and some forms of chemotherapy. Admittedly, there may be serious side effects as a consequence of undergoing these treatments. It must be acknowledged, however, that all medication, all forms of treatment, may have adverse effects; while being taken in an attempt to cure one illness, many treatments and medications may precipitate another illness. Even the little aspirin pill has caused serious troubles for some people.

How a patient reacts to varied treatments depends on many factors not the least of which is the general emotional and physical well being of the individual patient. I am pleased to say that I weathered my radiation therapy and chemotherapy treatments quite well and am hopeful that they brought about positive results internally.

I began my chemotherapy in January 1977 immediately after the surgery for my recurrence. This was as a safety precaution to destroy any cancer cells that may have wandered from the breasts to other areas of the body. I was told I would be on chemotherapy for ten months. Ten months later, in October 1977, I was told I had had enough and my chemotherapy was discontinued.

My radiation treatments took place during February and March and were completed on April 1, 1977. I am very much pro-radiation therapy. Thousands of cancer patients' lives have been saved by radiation therapy. Admittedly, most patients are to a lesser or greater degree frightened and/or traumatized as they lie on the "radiation table." While lying on this table, the patient feels nothing, sees nothing, smells nothing and tastes nothing of the gamma rays that are coming at her (or him). But, the patient knows that something serious is taking place, namely, that cobalt is being directed at the patient. If the patient has a positive attitude and knows the potential benefits of radiation therapy, the trauma is minimal. I believe time is precious, for time is life and, therefore, should not be wasted. So, I composed poetry as I was lying on the radiation table.

Weird occurrences continued to occur in the "weird world of breast cancer." Upon my return home from the hospital radiotherapy center after my first radiation treatment, I noted that the light was lit on my phone answering device. I rewound the cassette and then proceeded to listen to the messages. The first message was from a female caller.

A very affected female voice with an obviously "phony" accent said as follows: "Dr. Splaver, are you there?" _______ (pause) _______ "aw, shit, you're not there" _______ (pause) _______ "aw, I shit on you and your lumpectomy — goodbye — I'll call again."

And call again, she did. She called every single weekday, from Monday through Friday, until my final day of radiation therapy. Each time she left the same message. I do not know what this woman was trying to accomplish. But, I must admit that I got some good laughs from her and her weird message.

No one knows the cause(s) of breast cancer, but we do have some ideas. We do know that great stress has its physiological reverberations. I believe that my recurrence was caused in large part, if not entirely, by the tremendous unanticipated stress to which I was subjected by the many varied vile and vicious vested interests that want to perpetuate breast cancer, these interests that are angry because I had a lumpectomy rather than a mastectomy and because I came out of it all fighting against breast cancer — and many physicians agree with me!

I do not want anyone to misinterpret what I have said in the preceding paragraph. I am *not* saying that the emotions cause breast cancer. THE EMOTIONS DO NOT CAUSE CANCER, BREAST CANCER OR ANY OTHER CANCER. However, the emotions may be a secondary, precipitating factor. Additionally, if a breast cancer (or other cancer) patient is subjected to extremely stressful situations, especially from unexpected sources, recurrences may take place.

Had I know how much emotional abuse, harassment, humiliation and other vulgarities I would be subjected to by these many vested interests, had this all not come as such an incredible surprise, from such unanticipated sources, the stressful situations would have been less stressful for I would have been prepared for them.

Thus, I believe, I did not have a recurrence because I had local excision in July 1975. I had it because *breast cancer is the only illness that has so many vested interests that want to perpetuate that illness.* These vested interests were (and many still are) determined that the Breast Diseases Association of America should not be formed, should not exist, should not fight breast cancer.

It is over three years since I entered the "weird world of breast cancer." During this period of time, I have come to know more than 1,000 women who had mastectomies of all sorts. Many have told me the names of their surgeons and I have listened with great interest to their stories.

The truth should be known and it should be made known to the women of America — and the truth is — THE VERY SURGEONS, WELL KNOWN BREAST SURGEONS, who tell women that if they have local excision, they will suffer recurrences — MANY, MANY OF THEIR PATIENTS, PATIENTS ON WHOM THESE SURGEONS PERFORMED RADICAL SURGERY, HAVE SUFFERED RECURRENCES — RECURRENCES *6 MONTHS* and *8 MONTHS* and *12 MONTHS AFTER THEIR RADICAL SURGERY! These breast surgeons do not make these facts public!*

Many women who had local excision have *not* had recurrences although several years have passed since their surgery!

Not so long ago, I attended a breast cancer conference (among many I have attended) at which a well-known breast surgeon told an audience of physicians that all women who have a breast malignancy must have radical surgery, otherwise these women will suffer recurrences. I have met quite a number of women who had radical mastectomies performed on them by this same surgeon and many of them have told me of the recurrences they suffered within a year after the radical surgery performed on them by this well-known breast surgeon! WHY DID HE NOT TELL THE TRUTH!!!

May the good Lord have mercy on the women who may someday have a lump in their breast and may go to one of the physicians who sat in that auditorium and devoured the mistruths spouted by this well-known breast surgeon! It is a myth that *every* woman who has a breast malignancy must have a mastectomy — and this breast surgeon knows it! In private, I heard this same well-known misogynistic breast surgeon state that local excision (followed by radiation) is sufficient for those women whose malignancies are detected early!!!

During the Spring and Summer of 1977, several selfish, stupid and greedy people made attempts to destroy the Breast Diseases Association of America. BDAA weathered the storms, for the attempts of these people were so transparent. Had these attempts not been so disgraceful and outrageous, they would have been laughable.

On Tuesday, September 6, 1977, I went to my breast specialist for my periodic check-up which included mammography, thermography and clinical examinations. Happily, he said that all was well.

On November 9, 1977, the Breast Diseases Association of America became one year old and on Saturday, November 5th, it held its First Anniversary Luncheon in the Terrace Ballroom of the Hotel Roosevelt in New York City. Speakers brought greetings from the White House and the State House and the Mayor of the City of New York proclaimed the week of November 5th through 12th "Breast Diseases Association of America Week."

The Mayor's Proclamation states: "The Breast Diseases Association of America was formed a year ago to further education, research and improved patient care. The Association's objective is to reduce the incidence of breast diseases and lower death rates from breast cancer. The Association stresses early detection, effective treatment adapted to individual patient needs, including exploration of alternative methods of treatment, and psychological counseling beginning with initial diagnosis."

In the evening of Thursday, November 3rd — two days before the Luncheon — I received a threatening phone call. I had been receiving many calls as the Luncheon was approaching. Additionally, I had been on a radio program two days earlier and that resulted in many calls, a number of which were rather strange. Consequently, I did not pick up my phone receiver until the caller identified herself (or himself) in my phone answering device. This particular caller, in a well-modulated female voice, said, "Is Dr. Splaver there? I would like to speak with her."

I removed the receiver and said, "This is Dr. Splaver. May I help you?"

The caller said, "The Breast Diseases Association of America is having a First Anniversary Luncheon this Saturday." Then, she paused.

"Yes, that's correct," I said. And, then I asked, "Did you hear me on the air?"

The tone of the caller's voice changed as she said, "You'd better call off that Luncheon."

"No, we won't call it off. But, tell me, why should we call it off?" I asked.

She did not reply to my question. "I'm warning you. If you don't call off that Luncheon, when you get up to speak, I have a gun, and when you start to speak, I'll shoot you, and I'll guarantee you, you'll be dead."

Since the summer of 1975, when I announced that I had a tylectomy and that I was determined that there must be a national voluntary health association primarily concerned with breast diseases, especially breast cancer, I have received at least a dozen calls from disturbed women threatening to kill me, for they have vested interests in the perpetuation of breast cancer. The first call was upsetting, but I do not become frightened that readily. Thus, the calls that followed the first one, including this one, did not frighten me one bit.

I ignored what the caller said and asked her, "Are you a breast cancer patient?"

"None of your business," she growled.

"I am a breast cancer patient. I'd like to help you. Let's talk," I said.

"I'll shoot you. I guarantee you," she shouted.

"Why do you want to shoot me?," I asked, and then added, "Let's talk."

"When you start to speak, I guarantee you, I'll shoot you and you'll be dead," she shouted as she slammed the receiver down with a loud "bang."

I was convinced that this caller had no intention of shooting me, but was trying to unnerve me in an attempt to make the Luncheon unsuccessful. However, I do believe it is wise to play safe and, therefore, without telling him why, I asked the hotel banquet manager to have the speaker's lectern placed behind the dais rather than in front of it to give the speakers, including myself, greater protection. All went well. Nothing untoward happened. I told no one about this caller until the Luncheon was over.

Nothing angers some people as much as the success of other people. Thus, the success of BDAA's Luncheon brought tremendous anger to a cowardly man and two unscrupulous women who have vested interests in the perpetuation of breast cancer. As a result, certain outrageous acts took place after the Luncheon and throughout December 1977 and January 1978. This cowardly man and the two unscrupulous women made a massive attempt to "make trouble" for BDAA, an attempt to destroy BDAA. We used our minds and took the proper action. Consequently, they failed and I hope they have learned their lesson.

On Wednesday, March 1, 1978, I went to my breast specialist for my periodic mammography, thermography and clinical examinations. It was a delight to hear him say that all is well.

In May 1978, I received a phone call from the radiotherapy center of the hospital at which I had received my radiation treatments. My radiation therapist wanted me to come in to have my breasts photographed; the resulting slides would be used as part of a study he was preparing of breast cancer patients who had been treated at his center.

On Tuesday, May 16th, at 10:00 a.m., I arrived at the radiotherapy center for this photography. The "photographer" was a physician whom I had not met before. He adjusted his camera, looked at my breasts, and then asked me, "Which one is the breast that had the surgery and radiation?"

I was so pleased to hear this question. My left breast had been subjected to two lumpectomies and thirty radiation sessions and yet this physician was unable to tell the difference between my left breast and my right breast.

My next breast examination at the radiotherapy center had been scheduled for June. However, since I was at the hospital and it was already mid-May, the radiation therapist said it was perfectly all right to examine my breasts a bit ahead of schedule. After examining my breasts, he too said, as my breast specialist had said in March, that all is well.

Two days later, on Thursday, May 18, 1978, I had an appointment to have my breasts examined by my surgeon. This was an especially meaningful examination to me. A year and a half had passed from the time I was first stricken with breast cancer to the time of my recurrence. Now, it was a year and half since my recurrence. I prayed as my surgeon conscientiously examined my breasts. I heaved a sigh of relief and gave thanks to God when I heard my surgeon say, "Everything is all right."

Thank God, the wheel has hopefully begun to turn.

Months have passed since the last harassing phone call. The wheel has hopefully begun to turn here too and that brings great warmth and gratification to me.

I have never returned the vulgarities, obscenities and curses which have been hurled at me since I began my battle against breast cancer; this is not my nature. I shall never stoop to the depths of those who hurled this verbal filth at me. I did not — and never shall — permit them to pull me down to the gutter with them, though these be the gutters of some of New York's best streets.

Breast cancer is very much unlike any other illness and, therefore, there are many reasons why so many people want to perpetuate it. These reasons include: 1) breast cancer is big business, very big business, and many lust for money; 2) the mastectomy is a devastating surgical procedure that all too often leaves the mastectomee so mentally disordered that she wants all other women to be mastectomized too; and, 3) many have ulterior reasons too numerous to list.

To those who may wish to heave abuse on me because of something I have said in this book that they may not like or because of anything which I, with the help of many others, shall be doing to fight breast cancer, let me tell you a little tale that represents one of my basic philosophies of life.

When you do something different — to have local excision, to speak out in favor of lesser surgery for early breast cancer, and to be in some way instrumental in the formation of a health association to fight breast cancer are "something different" — your head sticks out above the crowd. When your head sticks out above the crowd, there are those who will throw tomatoes at you. I believe in catching those tomatoes, converting them into tomato juice, and having a nutritious, delicious drink.

My philosophy is: convert negatives into positives. With the inestimable help of my breast specialist and other friends, I have helped convert a negative — breast cancer — into a positive — the Breast Diseases Association of America. It has been good to hear many physicians say, "Keep it up. BDAA can only do good."

In all of these many decades in which thousands upon thousands of women had mastectomies performed on them, *why, oh why — I ask — did not one mastectomee — at least one among the many rich and famous mastectomees —* make an effort to form a Breast Diseases Association of America to fight breast cancer and all breast diseases?

I believe that if a Breast Diseases Association of America had been formed forty or thirty or twenty or perhaps even ten years ago, there is a good likelihood that breast cancer may, by now, have been conquered.

There was a National Tuberculosis Association years ago to fight tuberculosis. It won the fight. Tuberculosis is now a minor public health problem. There is no longer a National Tuberculosis Association. There is now an American Lung Association to fight such lung disorders as bronchitis, asthma, emphysema and other respiratory diseases. There was a National Infantile Paralysis Association to fight poliomyelitis (infantile paralysis). It won the fight. Polio has been conquered. There is no longer a National Infantile Paralysis Association; the March of Dimes (its subtitle) is now fighting to conquer birth defects.

I have been misquoted so many times by persons who have vested interests in the perpetuation of breast cancer that I want to state here, clearly and concisely, my views on the subject of the treatment of breast cancer. What I am going to say is based on all that I have read and heard and seen in three years of my immersion in and my intensive and extensive investigations of the "weird world of breast cancer," plus the totality of my educational and life's experiences.

1. *I am for early detection* because early detection followed by early treatment can not only save the woman's life, but may also spare her breasts.

2. *I am not against mastectomy* — where it is needed. When a mastectomy is needed, I believe the patient should be psychologically "prep"ed (in addition to surgical "prep"ing) for the mastectomy and she should receive psychological counseling before she leaves the hospital and for as long thereafter as supportive psychological counseling is deemed necessary.

3. *I am not for tylectomy* where the stage and state of the malignancy and other conditions preclude this mode of treatment.

4. *I am against breast cancer* — and I say it is time that we started to fight this battle in earnest. I am proud of the fact that a physician recently said to me, "BDAA is the only organization that is not playing games, that is determined to fight breast cancer."

5. Each case of breast cancer is different and each patient is different and, therefore, *the mode of treatment should match the individual case and the individual patient.*

6. *I want women to be informed of ALL the alternatives,* the gamut of all the modes of treatment available to them, if they are stricken with breast cancer.

7. I want women — in this great democracy of ours — to have the *FREEDOM TO CHOOSE from among all the alternatives that mode of treatment which best matches their individual case and their individual personality.*

8. *I believe women should consult with knowledgeable breast specialists* (not breast surgeons, but *breast specialists*) who will present them with options (alternatives) which will enable these women, with their *freedom of choice,* to choose, in partnership with their breast specialists, that alternative which best meets the needs of their individual case and their individual personality. The woman who consults first with a breast surgeon thereby chooses her mode of treatment — surgery — without permitting herself the freedom to choose from among all the alternatives; she is not being fair to herself.

9. *I believe physicians should treat the entire woman* — the entire person — and not just the breast cancer; we are total human beings and not just breasts.

I do not know how long I will live — nor does anyone else! But, my doctors and all of the other knowledgeable doctors I have met during the three years since I was first stricken with breast cancer tell me the prognosis in my case is excellent. I believe we stay on this earth for as long as the good Lord wishes us to stay. I am determined to stay and I am hopeful He will want me to remain here for a long time. Even when He does decide my time is up, I will probably resist and fight to stay, for I love life and I believe He has a lot of work for me to do right here on planet Earth.

My belief in God is as strong now as it was before I heard the words "it's malignant." Cancer of any variety is not caused by God. It is caused by people. We have polluted the air we breathe, the food we eat, and the water we drink — and these are now considered contributing causes for the increase in the number of cases of cancer. So, let us not blame God for our own stupidity!

I am glad I believe in God, for life is full of storms and the winds may sometimes howl at hurricane force as they surely do when you hear the words "it's malignant." God is a pillar of strength when the earth beneath us quakes. I'm glad He was there beside me when my "earth" was quaking in July 1975 and again at my recurrence in January 1977, for He with the aid of His superb assistants, my exceptional physicians — my breast specialist, my surgeon, my radiation therapist, and my family physician — have enabled me to continue to live a life of fulfillment with a minimal loss of time.

I have discussed the treatment of breast cancer with many oncologists. One oncologist recently said to me, "You've had your surgery — lesser surgery, and that's enough surgery. You've had radiation therapy and chemotherapy. Now, the thing to do is — PRAY."

A few days later, I told a second oncologist what this first oncologist had said. The second oncologist said he disagrees with the first one. He said, "From the moment you hear that you have a malignancy, you should start praying. Then, you have your surgery and you continue praying. Then, you have radiation therapy and you continue praying. Then, you have chemotherapy and you continue praying. And, you should continue praying for the rest of your life."

I agree with the second oncologist.

The Bible says, "A merry heart doeth good like a medicine."

I am convinced that the best "medicine" is "a merry heart," a positive attitude and positive outlook, and inner determination to get well — and, thank God, I have all of these.

God has been good to me. I am fortunate that my breast malignancy was detected early in July 1975 and again in January 1977. I am fortunate too to be treated by the best of the medical profession, a profession for which I have the highest regard despite the unhappy experiences I had with a small number of its members.

Now, with positve attitude and a deep determination to win the battle against breast cancer, I am looking forward to going forward for many, many malignancy-free years — years of fulfillment and of helping those less fortunate than myself — with the help of God and His brilliant assistant, my very knowledgeable and compassionate breast specialist.

Part Four

Breast Cancer is Curable

Come, Cooperate and Conquer it Completely

BREAST CANCER IS CURABLE
— COME, COOPERATE AND CONQUER IT COMPLETELY

You must make up your mind to become a partner with your breast specialist in the care and treatment of your breasts. This is on the individual, one to one, basis of physician and patient.

You must trust your physician and believe that what he (or she) is recommending to you is what he (or she) sincerely thinks is the best treatment for your specific condition. If you do not trust your physician, if you do not believe your physician is matching the treatment to your individual case, then you should find another physician.

In the conquest of breast cancer, you must also make up your mind to form a partnership, but a partnership on a larger scale. Women and men, physicians and surgeons, scientists and cancer researchers of all sorts must join together in an all-out war against breast cancer. The incidence of breast cancer is rising. The mortality rates are rising. This scourge must be stopped.

Before I was stricken with breast cancer, I knew a minimal number of women who had mastectomies. Since July 1975, I have come to know more than 1,000 mastectomees. I sympathize with their situations and would like to be of help to them. The mastectomee cannot help in the all-out war against breast cancer unless and until she is comfortable with herself.

The mastectomy is a devastating surgical procedure and it is normal for psychological problems to arise after such surgery. A woman needs a period of readjustment after a mastectomy. It is understandable that she will be depressed during a good part of this period.

The mastectomee is justified in being depressed, bitter, hostile and frustrated after her mastectomy. The breast is a very emotionally charged part of a woman's body. The woman who loses a breast (or both breasts) is generally emotionally traumatized. When a person has an amputation — and a mastectomy is an amputation — the emotions become entangled in this amputation.

Today, some women who had simple or modified radical mastectomies are having their breasts reconstructed; it is difficult, and often impossible, to perform breast reconstruction on those women who had radical mastectomies. Women who have had this reconstruction have told me they feel "whole" and "feminine" again. Increasing numbers of surgeons are telling their patients about this procedure. If the patients desire it, these surgeons invite the reconstruction surgeons to be present while the mastectomy is being performed. This makes it easier for the reconstruction surgeon to perform his surgery when he does it at an appropriate later date.

For the mastectomee to wallow in her woes for too long a while will be destructive and corrosive to her. Emotional tensions build if they are not released. It is best to direct them for release into wholesome channels, such as doing something constructive for oneself and others. If you are a mastectomee, you may ask how you, the mastectomee, can help yourself.

Yes, you can help yourself. You must learn to think in terms of what you have and not in terms of what you have not. In rehabilitation counseling, the popular dictum is: "It's what you have, and not what you don't have that counts. It's what you can do, and not what you can't do, that counts."

What has been done, has been done, and you must learn to accept it. You do not have two breasts. You have only one or perhaps none. This is not the worst of illnesses. It is not the worst of amputations. Accept what your surgeon told you, that this operation saved your life. And, now, you must go forward from here and consider what you do have — for, that's what counts! You must face reality with the will to conquer — to conquer your own cancer AND TO JOIN IN THE BATTLE TO CONQUER BREAST CANCER.

The emotionally healthy person learns to control her emotions and channels them into constructive, acceptable avenues. She dwells outside of herself, rather than within herself. She is people-oriented, rather than self-oriented. She considers the needs of others, rather than constantly thinking of "me-me-me."

To every mastectomee, I say: by becoming involved with others, by helping others, you will be helping yourself. As you help others, you will find that within you gratification will replace frustration, calm will replace fear, amiability will replace hostility, and kindness will replace bitterness. You will be on your way toward becoming a healthier person.

Count your blessings. There are millions of people less fortunate than yourself, despite your mastectomy. Get out of yourself — and help others — and you will become alive and content. Life will become meaningful. You will not need to say, "I am happier than I have ever been" and know within you that you are telling an untruth. When you stop concentrating on yourself and start thinking of helping others and actually start to help others less fortunate than yourself, then you will be able to say, "I am happy," and it will be the truth.

There is a question I would like to ask every mastectomee: why do you refer to yourself as a "mastectomee"? I have used this term in this book because that is the way you refer to yourself. It indicates a very negative self-image. You not only defeminize yourself in this manner, you even depersonalize yourself.

If you had your appendix removed, would you refer to yourself as an "appendectomee"? If you had your gall bladder excised (a surgical procedure known as a "cholecystectomy"), would you call yourself a "cholecystectomee"? Sounds ridiculous, doesn't it? Then, why do you refer to yourself as a "mastectomee"? You are a *woman* who had a mastectomy! You are a *woman*, first and foremost, and you happened to have a mastectomy.

Start thinking of yourself in positive terms — and positive thoughts will lead to positive acts!

In the war against cancer, as in any war, we must first face the enemy. If we cannot face it, how will we vanquish it? The enemy is *cancer*, not "Ca" or "big C." These terms represent flight from reality. They were, perhaps, suitable in the past when just about nothing was known about cancer. Today, approximately

2,000,000 persons, who at one time had cancer, are alive and living active, productive lives.

So, we must make up our minds to face the enemy. If we face it, we won't fear it. Enough of yesterday's fright and flight from reality. Today is the time for fight, not fright.

Illness is equivalent to receiving a "knockout" blow. You are down. But, you must not stay down. Some blows — like cancer — are harder to take than others and that makes it difficult to get up. But, get up one must! Get up and with cheerful attitude, positive outlook and inner determination fight your malignancy in specific; then, make up your mind to fight malignancy in general.

We must all make up our minds to become partners in the conquest of breast cancer for everyone is vulnerable. With the concentrated efforts and cooperation of everyone — breast specialists, surgeons, radiation therapists, chemotherapists, medical oncologists, physicians of all sorts, cancer researchers, breast cancer patients (regardless of their modes of treatment), and men and women from all walks of life — breast cancer can be conquered completely and discussions about mastectomy will be academic rather than epidemic.

Although they are all essentially different, there is reason to believe that there is a basic common denominator among all cancers. When we find the cause(s) and cure for breast cancer, we will surely begin to find the answers to all cancers.

Come, cooperate in the battle to conquer breast cancer so that no women — or men — will ever again lose their lives or their breasts to this scourge. Let's make up our minds to fight breast cancer on the individual small scale and on the large overall scale.

Breast cancer is curable and with concerted cooperation we can conquer it completely in this country and throughout the world.

If I can stop one heart from breaking
I shall not live in vain
If I can ease one life the aching
Or cool one pain

Or help one fainting robin
Unto his nest again
I shall not live in vain.

Emily Dickinson

ATTENTION:
ALL WHO HAD LESSER SURGERY

Are you a breast cancer patient who was treated by lesser surgery (lumpectomy, biopsy followed by radiation therapy, or any other mode of treatment which enabled your breast to remain intact)?

If you are, I would be grateful to you if you would write to me. There is a paucity of statistics on the women who had lesser surgery. In many cities and states, no central records are kept of breast cancer patients whose mode of treatment was lesser surgery, with the possible exception of those patients who had radiation therapy at a recognized radiation therapy center following such surgery.

On the basis of my investigations and conversations with breast specialists, surgeons, radiation therapists and other oncologists, it is apparent that there are thousands of breast cancer patients throughout the country who had lesser surgery and whose breasts are intact. These women are alive and living active, productive lives years after their lesser surgery. Knowledgeable breast specialists, surgeons, radiation therapists and other oncologists accept the fact that lesser surgery is an effective mode of treatment for early breast cancer. The time has come for the entire medical profession and all people to know and accept this fact.

I have spoken with many women who, like myself, had lesser surgery. When I asked them to speak up, some of them replied, "Look at the harassment you have had to endure because you spoke up. We don't want that harassment." So, many of them have remained "in the closet" just as most women who had mastectomies have done for lo these many years. My reply is that there would be little, if any, harassment if all breast cancer patients who chose not to have mastectomies would proudly proclaim this fact.

A woman who had a mastectomy recently said to me, "If women who had lumpectomies would say so and if people would get to know that if you have breast cancer it doesn't necessarily mean you must lose your breast, this would be a big service to all the women who had mastectomies. Then, if we would tell people we had breast cancer, they would wonder — did she or didn't she — lose her breast — instead of taking it for granted that we did."

No one — woman or man — need be ashamed of having breast cancer. It is an illness, just as diabetes and pneumonia and ulcers and hypertension — and so on ad infinitum — are illnesses. All breast cancer patients — and all people — must join in the battle against breast cancer. Those of us who chose lesser surgery as our mode of treatment can play especially significant roles in this battle.

If you had lesser surgery, please write to me at the following address: Dr. Sarah Splaver, VERITAS PRESS, 3310 Rochambeau Ave., New York, N.Y. 10467.

Thank you.

Sarah Splaver, Ph.D.

Not the

End

but the

Beginning

of

The Battle Against

Breast Cancer

About the Author

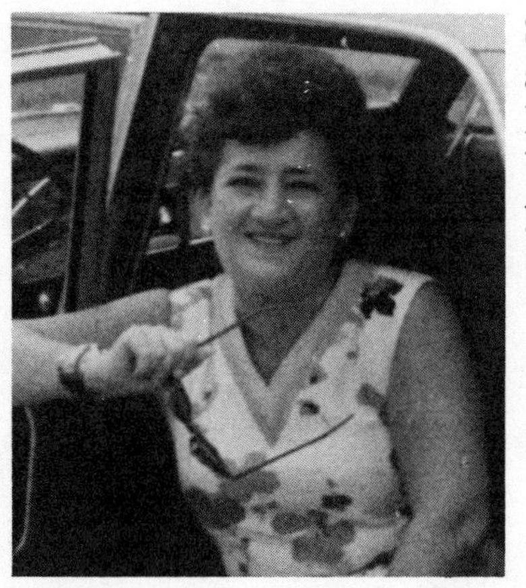

SARAH SPLAVER is a noted counseling and consulting psychologist. She holds a Doctor of Philosophy degree from New York University. She served for several years as a high school director of guidance. She became nationally and internationally well known as the originator of the socio-guidrama, a group guidance technique used as a means of helping young people with their problems.

Dr. Splaver is certified as a psychologist by the Department of Education of the State of New York. She has served as a consultant on psychological and guidance projects to the U.S. Defense Department, Department of the Army; U.S. Department of Health, Education and Welfare; International Business Machines Corp.; New York Life Insurance Company; and varied other organizations.

She has written many books in the fields of guidance and psychology. Her articles have appeared in professional journals and other publications. Dr. Splaver has lectured at conferences, conventions, young people's gatherings, and parent-teacher and other meetings. She has counseled thousands of young people and adults and now is counseling cancer patients.

Dr. Splaver is a Life Member of the American Personnel and Guidance Association. Among the other professional associations in which she holds membership are the American Psychological Association, American Rehabilitation Counseling Association, American School Counselor Association, American Association for the Advancement of Science, International Council of Psychologists, National Vocational Guidance Association, and the Authors Guild.

Dr. Splaver holds a certificate as a Health Service Provider in Psychology issued by the Council for the National Register of Health Service Providers in Psychology. She is also listed in *Who's Who of American Women, Who's Who in the East,* and *Who's Who in America.*